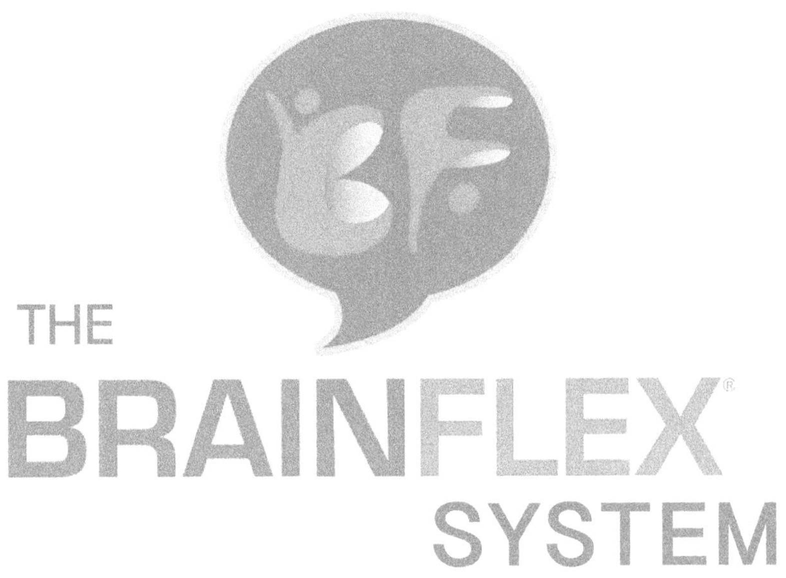

The Whole Person
Approach to Brain Health

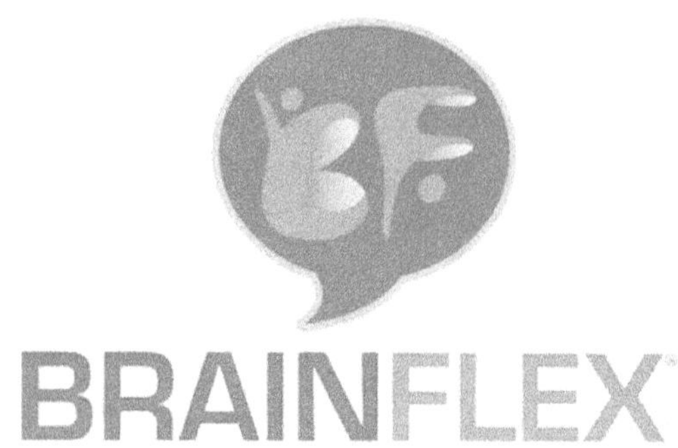

Volume 2 of 12 from 'The EARLY MILD Series'
For those who want to be proactive against age related diseases, including those that cause cognitive impairment.

www.brainflexwellness.com

Workbook Table of Contents

Welcome to The BRAINFLEX System!

Congratulations! You've just taken another step in keeping your brain healthy for life!

The BrainFlex System makes maintaining the brain fun and easy. But don't be fooled by the fun! BrainFlex activities incorporate the lessons of medical research to keep the brain as healthy as possible while seniors age or face illnesses that impact the brain.

Each BrainFlex lesson includes 5 key components that work together to give the brain just what it needs each day to stay in top form.

Brain Exercise: Use it or lose it! Included in each of the 8 lessons are 3-5 brain stimulating exercises, all designed to stimulate various areas of the brain. Activities focus on creativity, problem solving, self-expression, brainstorming, etc., while others require a more structured focus requiring a more analytical or logical approach, and there are plenty of opportunities to exercise areas of the brain related to reasoning and math as well. Last, a life-long learning component (new information) is also incorporated into each workbook, which is designed to increase the brain's cognitive reserve.

Socialization: Whether seniors enjoy doing the workbook with others, or alone, our unique *'Discussion Sheets'* open the door for conversation at any time. Every lesson includes one BrainFlex *"News You Can Use"* sheet, focusing on a wide range of important topics, including the 'why' behind our BrainFlex concepts. Other topics include mental and emotional self-care, the importance of healthy sleep patterns, the impact of a positive mindset, healthy communication, tips on how to keep your relationships strong, and more! Each *'Discussion Sheet'* is designed to inform, educate, and encourage conversation.

Welcome to The BRAINFLEX System!

Nutrition: We are what we eat! Our goal is to stay mindful of the impact food choices have on the brain and body, as well as one's over-all well-being, and according to research, the healthier the gut, the healthier the brain. Four recipes are included in each workbook. Recipes are carefully selected and crafted for ease of preparation and enjoyment while eating! Nutritional information in the primary ingredients and specific benefits for the brain and body are listed with each recipe.

Physical Exercise/Meditation/Prayer:

Physical Exercise: Research tells us that physical activity is THE MOST IMPORTANT way to keep the brain healthy. Each workbook includes a monthly guide with detailed written and visual instructions, covering a variety of stretching and strengthening exercises. The goal of the exercise guide is to increase and/or maintain range of motion, strengthen the core and other vital muscles, increase oxygen flow and heart rate, (safely), and boost coordination, while reinforcing the brain-body connection.

Meditation/Prayer: Research confirms chronic stress ages the brain. It has also been shown that our 'mindset' impacts both the brain and body, making thinking and speaking positively vital to 'aging well'. Each BrainFlex workbook incorporates a variety of techniques, including breathing exercises, to help develop strategies to keep worry and anxiety away. Workbooks also include an instruction guide for prayer/meditation and a list of self-affirmations are included in each lesson.

To help seniors stay on track, workbooks in 'The Prevention' and 'Early-Mild' series' include a 'Personal Action Plan', which allows seniors to set monthly goals for each of the BrainFlex concepts.
(Brain Stimulation, Socialization, Nutrition and Exercise w/Prayer and Meditation.)
'Wellness Notes' are provided to track the progress of each goal.

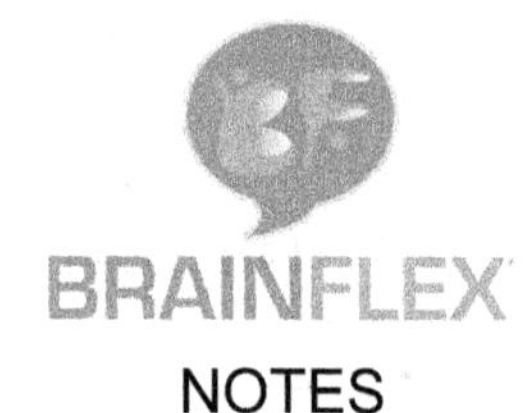

NOTES

few notes from the experts...

Tips for Successful Aging by Rosemary Laird, MD

1.) Stay Sharp!

Keeping mentally sharp as we age is something we all want. No one wants to lose the independence that comes with a sound mind. While genetic predisposition controls some of how our brains age, there are several key areas we can control that can help our brains stay healthy and keep those senior moments at bay.

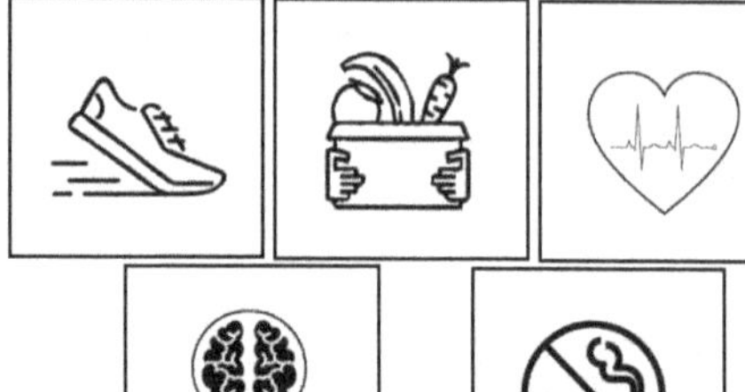

- Get 30 minutes of moderate physical activity each day

- Keep blood pressure and blood sugar in the normal ranges

- Follow the MIND and/or Mediterranean diets

- Keep cognitively active – be a lifelong learner and stay engaged in life

- Don't smoke

2.) Steady as You Go!

One of the earliest signs of a body slowing down and aging is when muscles become weak. When weakness affects the legs, an individual will find it harder to get up out of their chair. They will spend more of each day sitting and become less mobile. This will lead to lower endurance and decreased overall ability to walk, which then makes them weaker, and the continuous downward spiral is set. This weakness also increases the risk of falls and injury which only adds to the decline in ability.

One of the best ways to avoid this is to keep moving and plan 30 minutes of a moderately rigorous activity each day. Move it or lose it is very true!

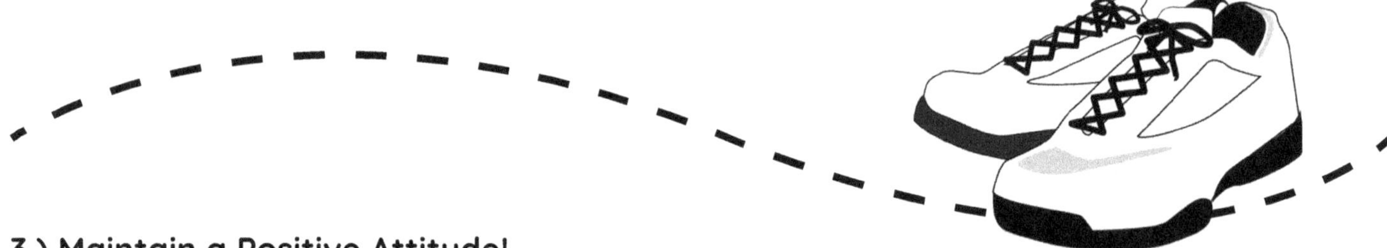

3.) Maintain a Positive Attitude!

Keeping a positive attitude as you get older may seem like a tall order, but it has a big payout. Research has shown a direct correlation between a positive attitude about aging during midlife being linked to people with delays in some of the common changes of aging such as cognitive decline, heart problems, and longevity. Other research has shown that a positive attitude is related to lower overall stress levels and that leads to a healthier state for your mind and body, so smile and remember "It's all in your head."

Scan the QR code with your phone camera to view another resource about maintaining a positive mindset.

Dr. Rosemary Laird's Tips to Successful Aging

4.) Stay Self-Assured Through It All!

Adaptation and resilience are two key attributes to aging successfully. Being able to adapt to changes in your body can mean the difference between continuing to thrive or starting down a path of decline. Here are two examples of common age-related conditions that could negatively impact your daily quality of life unless you keep a positive mindset and learn all you can about how to adapt.

- Hearing loss: Don't get left out of the conversation! Staying engaged and involved with others is a key component of healthy and successful aging. Hearing loss is one of the most common age-related challenges we all face to some degree. If it begins to impact your ability to interact with others, that's a strong indication that you need to seek help. If you answer YES to any of the following questions please schedule an appointment for a hearing evaluation:

  1) Are you having hearing problems when visiting with family and friends?
  2) Do you fear meeting new people due to a hearing problem?
  3) Does a hearing problem cause you to have arguments with family or friends?

- Urinary incontinence: Don't miss the party! This is perhaps the most embarrassing of the changes that can come as we age. We get it, we really do! The good news is there is often a lot you can do to reduce urinary incontinence and manage it discreetly. Don't let this get you down. Make an appointment to talk with your primary care provider or gynecologist. Also, check out the Seni website, www.seni-usa.com. You will find helpful information about what causes urinary incontinence, what to talk to your doctor about, and strategies and products you can use to help keep urinary incontinence from causing you to miss out on life.

Scan the QR code to learn more!

This pro-**active** approach will help you face and adapt to the common challenges of aging.

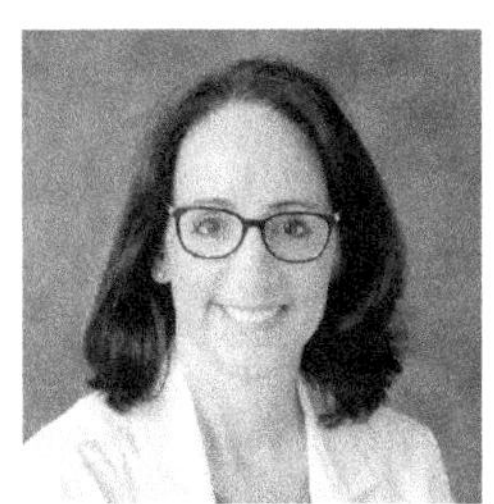

Rosemary Laird, M.D., M.H.S.A is a Clinical Associate Professor in the Department of Geriatrics at the Florida State University School of Medicine. Dr. Laird also now serves as a Principal Investigator for ClinCloudResearch in Viera, Florida.

Dr. Laird received her medical degree with honors from Georgetown University School of Medicine in 1991. She completed an Internal Medicine residency and Geriatric Fellowship. She is a recognized expert in diagnosing and caring for patients with Alzheimer's disease and spent 20 years as the Medical Director for two state-designated Memory Disorder Clinics. In 2019, the governor of Florida appointed her to serve on the state's Alzheimer's Disease Advisory Committee.

Dr. Laird is a sought-after speaker, educator, author and named the American Geriatrics Society's Geriatrician of the Year in 2013. She has guided the development of educational programs for lay and professional audiences, covering various topics related to Alzheimer's disease, other common conditions of aging, and family caregiving. She is a passionate advocate for the support of family caregivers and co-authored the book *Take Your Oxygen First: Preserving Your Health and Happiness While Caring for a Loved One with Alzheimer's Disease*. Dr. Laird is also a co-author with the late Fred Lee of *Beyond Disney: Heartwiring Healthcare Excellence*. She speaks to healthcare providers about this novel approach of infusing the heart of medical practice into the challenging world of clinical medicine.

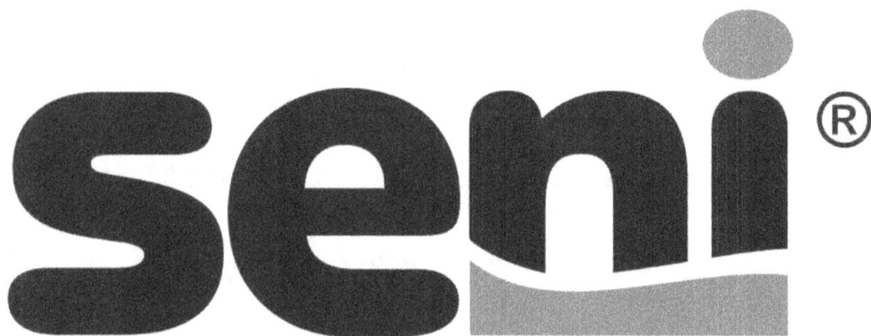

We want to thank our sponsor, Seni®, for their contribution to the *Aging Well* journey! As international experts in managing the challenges of urinary incontinence, Seni® shares our *whole person* philosophy and understands how the many physical changes of aging and common illnesses can have a tremendous impact on independence and overall quality of life. If there comes a time when incontinence holds you back, you can have confidence in turning to Seni®.

Your brain will thank you!

To Find the Right Product, Think **seni**®

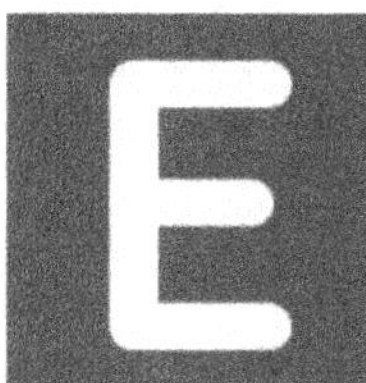

S is for Size

Waist/Hip measurement is important. Weight will not give sufficient information to determine the right size

*if measurements are in one range, pick the size this range indicates

*If measurements are in two different ranges, defer to the larger size.

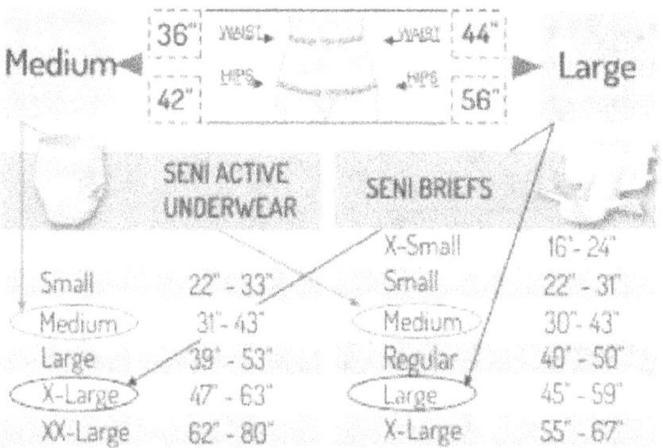

	SENI ACTIVE UNDERWEAR		SENI BRIEFS	
Small	22" - 33"	X-Small	16" - 24"	
Medium	31" - 43"	Small	22" - 31"	
Large	39" - 53"	Medium	30" - 43"	
X-Large	47" - 63"	Regular	40" - 50"	
XX-Large	62" - 80"	Large	45" - 59"	
		X-Large	55" - 67"	

E is for Essential Features, Evaluate Mobility, and Ensure Correct Style

Essential Features:

 Fully Breathable Outer Layer

Superabsorbency

Hydrophobic Standing Side Gathers

Extra Dry System - soft non-woven layer

Evaluate Mobility

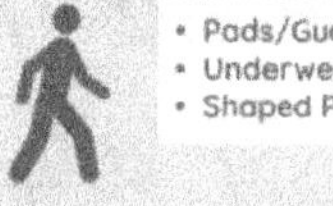

- Pads/Guards
- Underwear
- Shaped Pads

- Briefs
- Shaped Pads

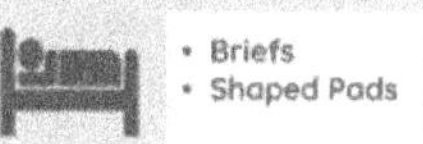

- Briefs
- Shaped Pads

Ensure Correct Style

Pads, Active Underwear, and Shaped Pads Day are ideal for someone with light to moderate incontinence. High Absorbency Underwear, Briefs, & Shaped Pads Night are ideal for someone with heavy/severe incontinence

ⓘ Underwear is a better style for dementia patients because they look and feel more like regular undergarments

ⓘ Man Fit guards are ideal for after prostate surgery

ⓘ Shaped pads are ideal for bariatric patients or those who fall in between sizes

N is for Night vs. Day Products

Sleep is valuable. Restorative sleep will help reduce the risk of falls at night and help you be more alert during the day.

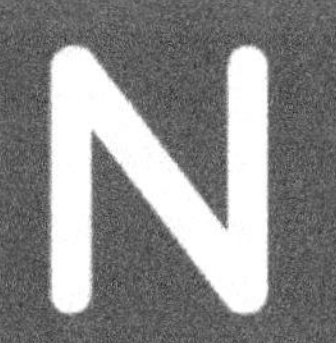

For daily use, choose products that are comfortable, easy to change, and at the right absorbency level.

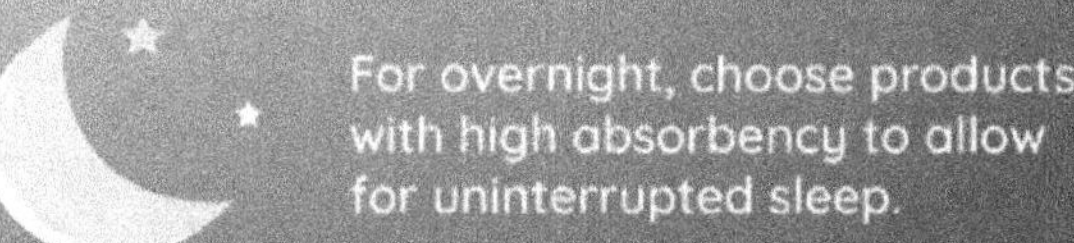

I is for Improve your Continence whenever Possible

See what other factors may influence each person's individual product assessment.

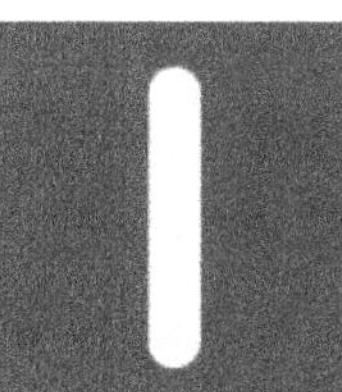

Avoid blockages to and from the bathroom. Adjust the environment for easy access.

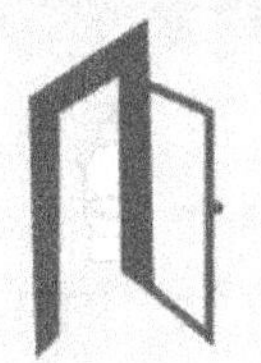

Recommend or perform Kegel exercises to strengthen pelvic floor muscles.

Create a personalized toileting schedule

www.seni-usa.com

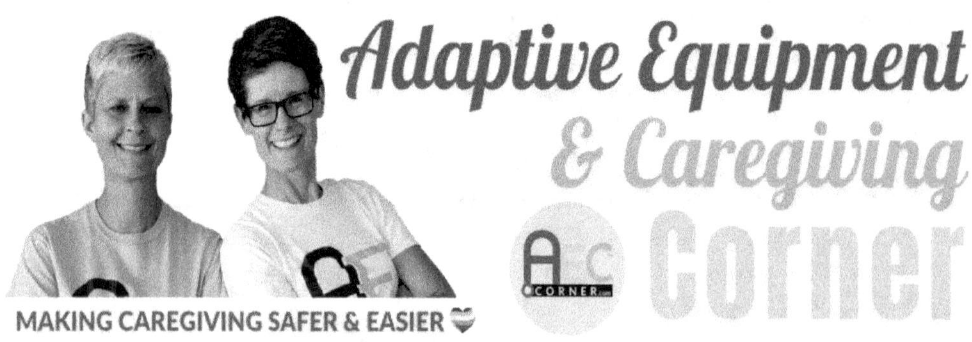

We show you how to safely care for someone

Easy-to-Understand Videos
Helpful Caregiver Tips
Links to Senior Service Resources

Want access to AECorner's premium video library?
We have two plans available:
The Caregiver Plan = $9.99/month
    Individual Access
The Company Plan = $100.00/month
    Group Access

AECorner's Caregiver Support video collection shows individuals how to stay safe in the home, wherever they call home and educates caregiver on ways to keep their loved ones and themselves safe while giving care.

Adaptive Equipment
& Caregiving
Corner

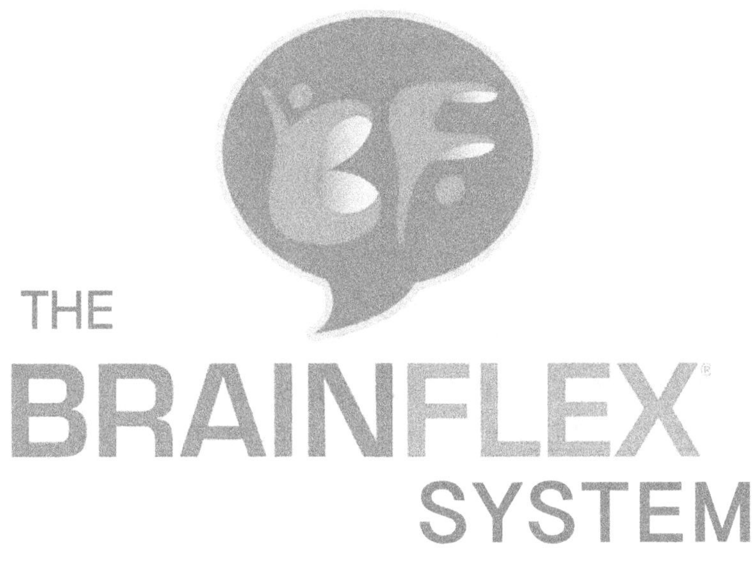

WORKBOOK GUIDE

This workbook is designed to
be used in a variety of settings.

1. Small Groups
2. One on One
3. Individually

THE BRAINFLEX SYSTEM WORKBOOK GUIDE

The purpose of this guide is to help the user navigate through the workbook successfully, which will ensure everyone involved experiences the very best outcomes.

There are three categories for which the workbooks in the BrainFlex System were designed.

1. <u>Small Groups:</u>
     a. Independent Living
     b. Assisted Living
     c. Adult Day Programs
     d. Senior Centers, Church Groups, Etc.
2. <u>Family or hired caregivers</u>: (working one on one with seniors)
3. <u>Seniors working independently</u>

The BrainFlex System includes a three different series of interactive workbooks, each packed with brain stimulating activities that go beyond typical brain games and is the most comprehensive aging well program available in this format.

There are three levels in 'The BrainFlex System' series of workbooks.

1. The 'Prevention' Series
     a. This workbook series consists of volumes 1 through 12, with each workbook designed to last one month, (2 lessons per week), and is appropriate for the following:
          i. Anyone who would like to take a preventative (proactive) approach to aging well and brain health.
2. The 'Early ~ Mild' Series. (For those in the early stages of MCI)

     a. This workbook series consists of volumes 1 through 12, and is appropriate for those who have been experiencing dementia but can still understand and follow directions.
          i. Anyone experiencing mild memory loss but is determined to do all they can do to slow this process down.

          ii. Anyone who may be in the early stages of Alzheimer's or one of the other diseases that impacts brain function and would like to maintain their brain and/or slow the decline.

3. The 'Mid ~ Moderate' Series: For those w/Alzheimer's (and related diseases)
    a. This workbook series consists of volumes 1 through 12, with each workbook designed to last one month. (2 sessions/week) and is appropriate for those who may have been experiencing dementia for some time but can understand and follow basic directions with visual or verbal cuing.

The BrainFlex System has been developed for seniors committed to aging well, which is why each workbook is focused on 'the whole person'. This includes the brain, body, mind, spirit, emotions, and relationships. According to research, engaging in activities that contribute to the health of these areas is what gives seniors the best chance to maintain independence. Each concept of the BrainFlex program encourages seniors to be proactive against age related diseases, including Alzheimer's. 'The BrainFlex Workbook' equips seniors with the tools needed to age well.

The interactive lesson plans are designed to be completed in one month, (2 lessons each week). Each lesson takes 2 to 3 hours to complete in a group setting, and about 1 ½ to 2 hours if done alone or with one other person.

NOTE: Sessions can be broken up into 2, 3 or 4 smaller sessions throughout the day or completed in one fun-filled session. *(i.e. Exercise @ 9am, Brain Stimulating Activities @ 11am, Interactive Nutrition @ 2pm and Meditation/Prayer with Self-Affirmations @ 7pm)* With that being said, our experience doing this live is that seniors enjoy the 2½ to 3 hour sessions.

KEEP IN MIND:
It's important to complete each worksheet in the lesson, rather than skipping around to find the activity that's most enjoyable. Although we understand this temptation ☺, it will not provide exercise to every area of the brain. As a matter of fact, the activities you enjoy the least are likely to be the most beneficial to your brain.

Both The Preventative Series and The Early ~ Mild Series of workbooks include a 'Personal Action Plan'. This plan is created by the individual, (although family members and/or caregivers may also want to contribute), and is based on the four concepts that have been shown to contribute the most to 'Aging Well' and to help slow down cognitive decline. Two goals are created for each of the <u>concepts</u> on which the BrainFlex program is built. *(See these concepts on the following page.)*

BrainFlex Concepts

1. Social |Connections
2. Nutrition
3. Brain Stimulating Activities
4. Physical Exercise with Meditation

(A positive mindset and healthy sleep patterns are also key to aging well and discussed frequently throughout the workbooks.)

Tracking your Monthly Personal Action Plan:
Steps taken to meet goals on the personal action plan can be tracked on the weekly 'Wellness Journal' pages, found in the back of each workbook in the 'Preventive' and 'Mild/Early' series'. The 'Personal Action Plan' and the 'Wellness Notes' are wonderful tools for families and primary care physicians.

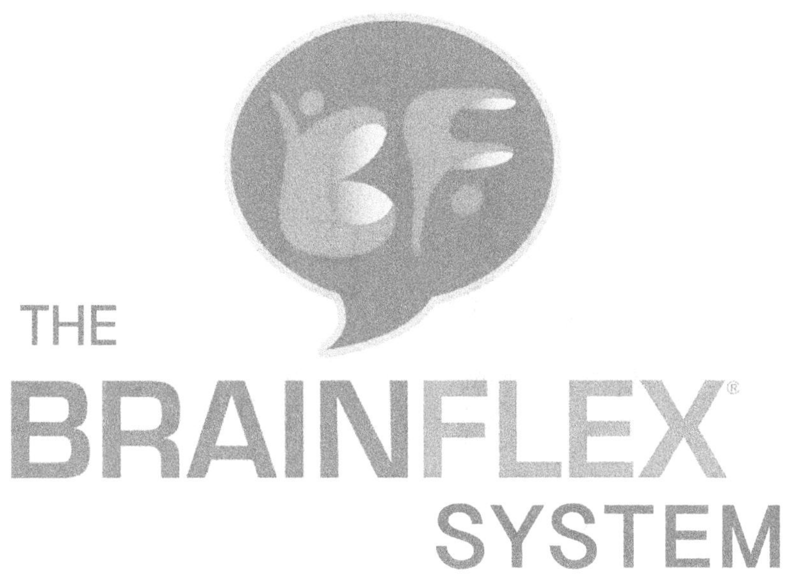

The Whole Person
Approach to Brain Health

EXERCISE
FOR OPTIMUM
BRAIN HEALTH

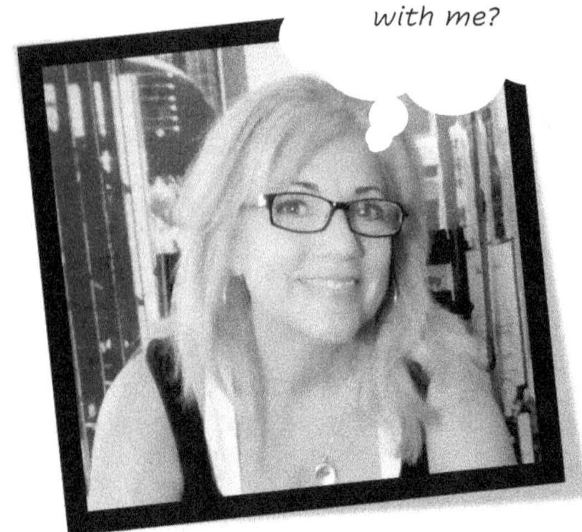

Exercise Series

You should always speak to a doctor before you change, start or stop any part of your healthcare plan, including physical activity or exercise.

Also, be sure to speak with your doctor before exercising if the following are applicable to you:

1. A long period of inactivity
2. Recent hospitalization
3. Recent surgeries

Stop and call 911 if you experience the following:

1. Unexplained shortness of breath
2. Pain in your neck, shoulders or arms
3. Leg pain, with or without swelling or tenderness
4. Dizziness
5. No one knows your body like you, so be sure to report
         anything that feels abnormal or unusual

IMPORTANT REMINDERS:
1. Form is very important. Be sure to keep your core tight, as if you are pulling your belly button back towards your spine.

2. Unless the exercise specifically instructs otherwise, keep your chin up, your shoulders back, and ensure your spine is as straight as possible. *(Avoid doing anything that causes you pain.)*

3. If at all possible, avoid using the back of the chair for support during exercise. Doing so will keep you from engaging your core, which is **KEY to balance**.

4. Take breaks when necessary, and be sure to drink plenty of water, before...during and after exercise.

Neck Stretch

Counting to 10, slowly begin to tilt your head so the ear is over the shoulder as shown below. Follow the visual guide, hold for 5 seconds and count to 10 as you raise your head back to the starting position.
Repeat the stretch on the opposite side.

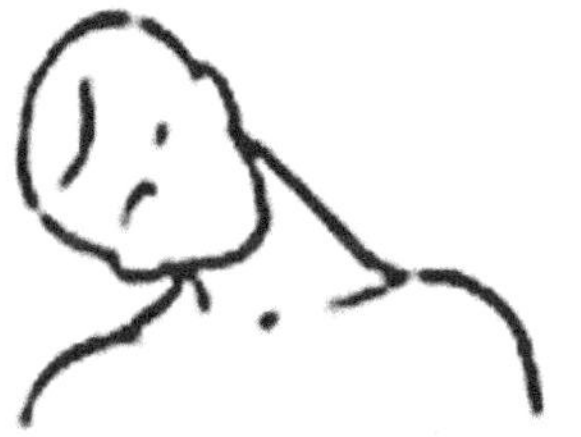
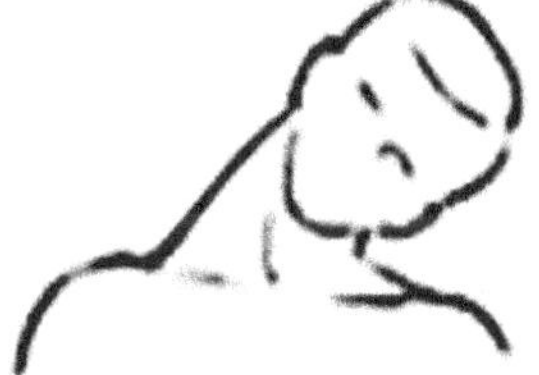

Remember:
Refrain from doing anything that causes pain.

Hand, Finger and Arm Stretches

Follow the visual guide to begin stretching the muscles in your arms, hands & fingers, very gently. While counting to 10, gently lift the arms gently above the head.
(It's okay if you aren't able to lift arms straight up.)

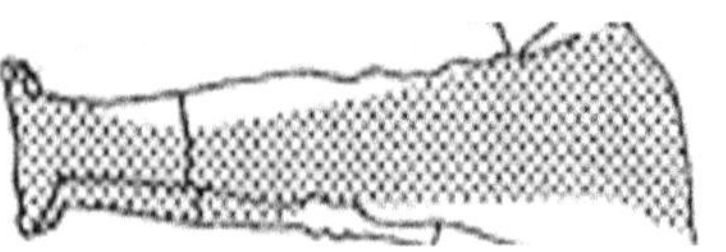

While counting to 10, slowly bring the arms back down,
then repeat for one more stretch.

Remember: Refrain from doing anything that causes pain.

The Shoulder Shrug

Follow the visual guide to begin slowly stretching your neck and shoulder muscles, very gently.

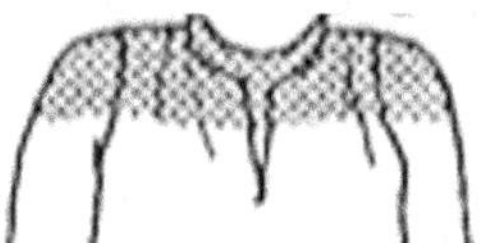

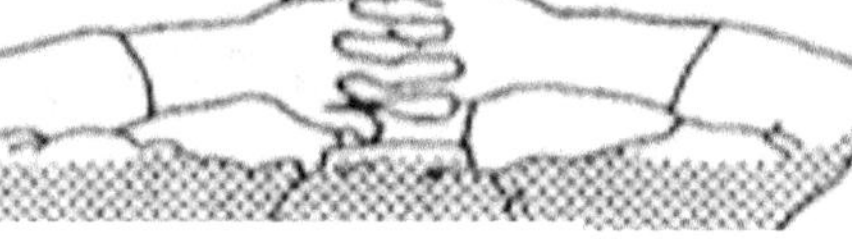

The Pectoral Stretch

Complete a total of 8 shoulder shrugs and
1 pectoral stretch,
(If you're able to do so.)

Total Arm Exercises

Lift your arms, bending them at the elbow to make a 90-degree angle. Using your body's resistance, bring them together, in front of your face, while keeping the arms at the same angle, then return back to the starting position, allowing your elbows to open as wide as possible.
(Remember: refrain from doing anything that causes you pain and/or discomfort.)

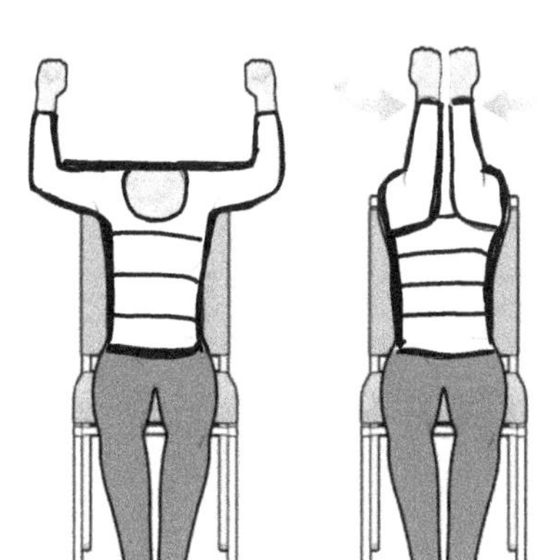

Complete 12 to 16 sets

Seated March

Sit up straight and imagine that an invisible string is pulling your belly button back towards your spine.
(For a strong core, try to hold this posture.)
Begin lifting your knees, one at a time, toward the ceiling, in an emphasized march

March for 2 minutes or as endurance allows.

(Put on some upbeat music, and this will quickly turn into a fun cardio exercise!)

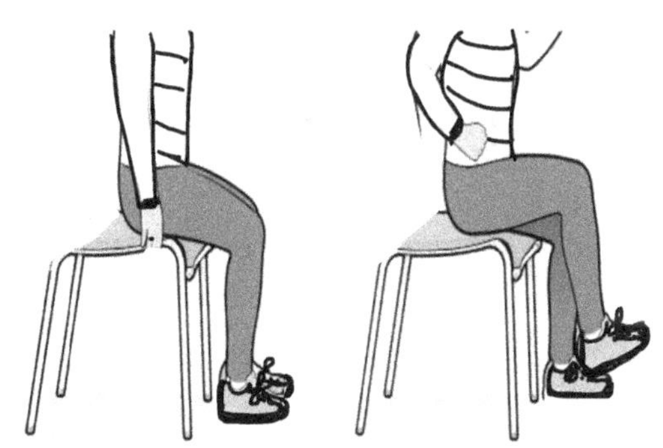

Core and Leg Workout

Begin sitting straight up, with your belly button pulled into your spine. This helps strengthen the core.

This exercise includes 4 slides with written and visual instructions. This is slide 1 of 4.

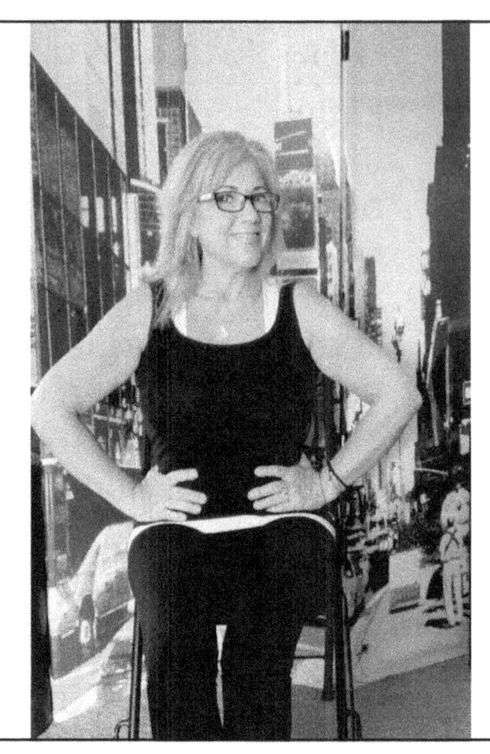

Start the exercise by lifting one knee straight up (towards the ceiling), Remembering to keep your core nice and tight...

Slide 2 of 4

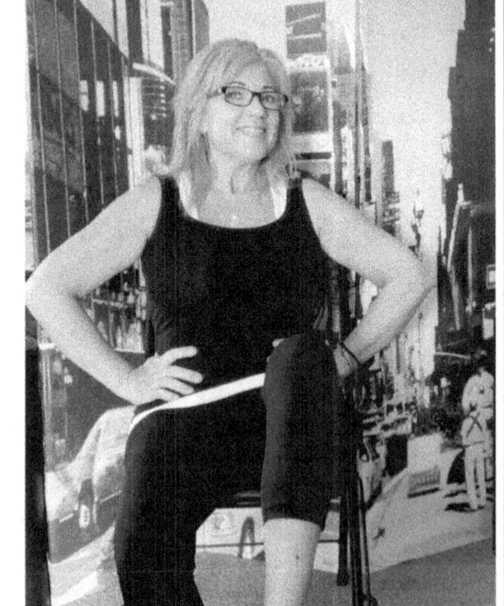

Continue by lifting the leg up, over and out, then barely tap the toe, before lifting the leg straight up and back to the starting position.

Slide 3 of 4

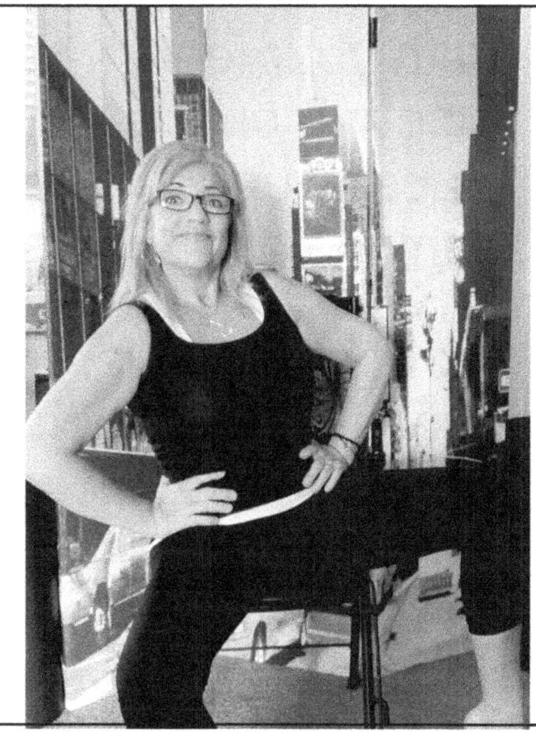

Once you return to the starting position,
(as if you were lifting your leg over a fire),
do the same exercise on the opposite leg.

Alternate legs,
24 repetitions.
(12 on each side.)

Slide 4 of 4

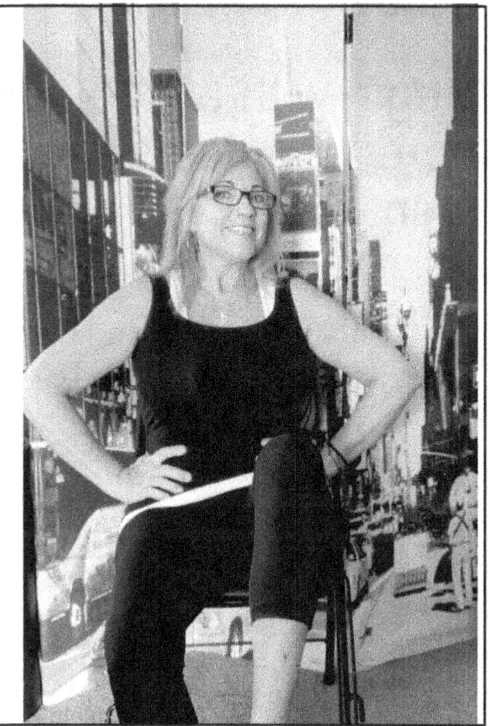

Waist and Core Exercise

With your feet together on the floor, place your hands behind your head.
(if comfortable)
Slowly turn toward the right, twisting at the waist, then return to the starting position, and repeat, twisting to the left.

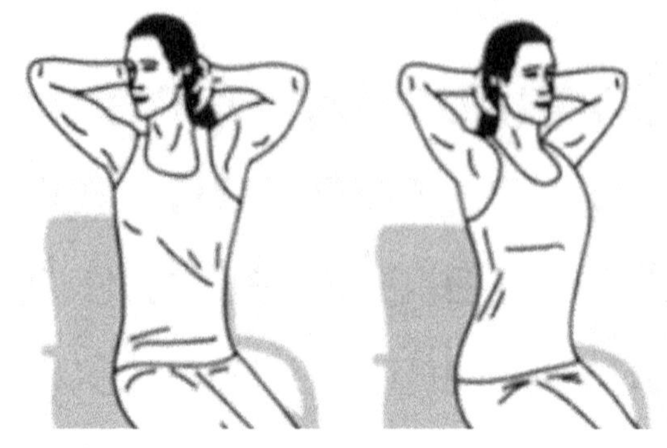

Complete 10 sets.

Thigh Exercises

Begin with a nice and tight core, shoulders back, and chin up.

Lift the right leg, until it's completely extended, hold for 10 seconds.

Repeat with opposite leg.

Complete one set of 8.
(8 lifts on each side.)

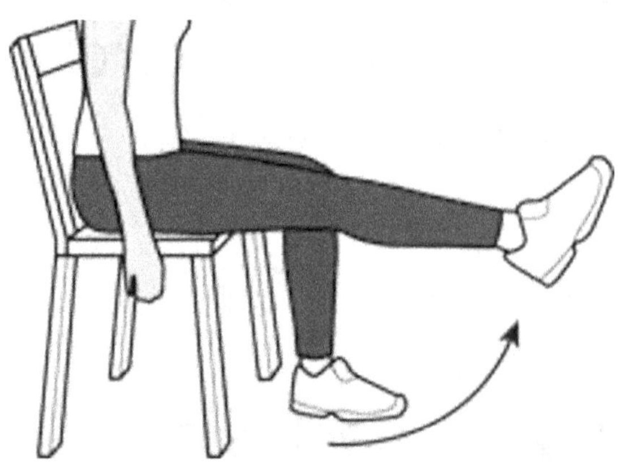

Arm Exercises

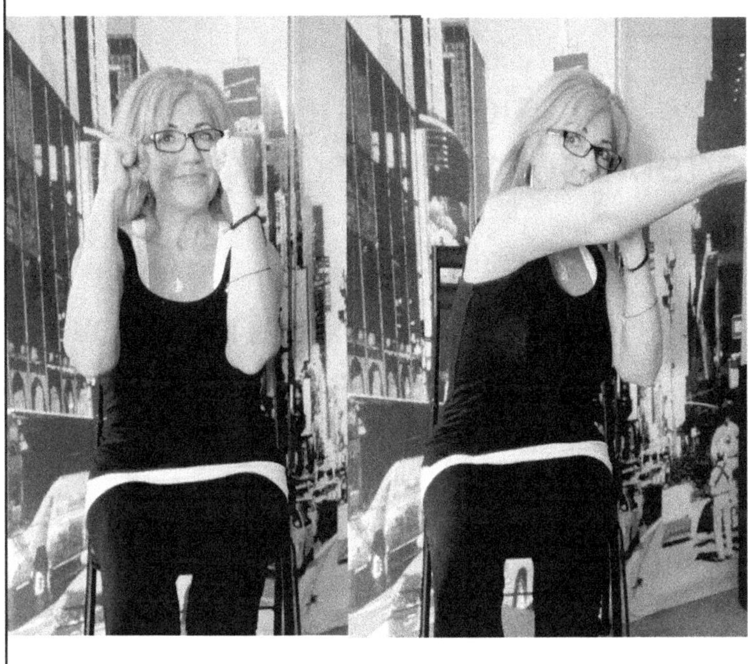

<u>Cross Body Jab (1 of 2)</u>

Plant your feet, and place your arms in a 'guarded' position.

Begin with a cross body jab using your right arm. Be sure to include a slight twist at the waist. Quickly return to the starting position.

(continued below)

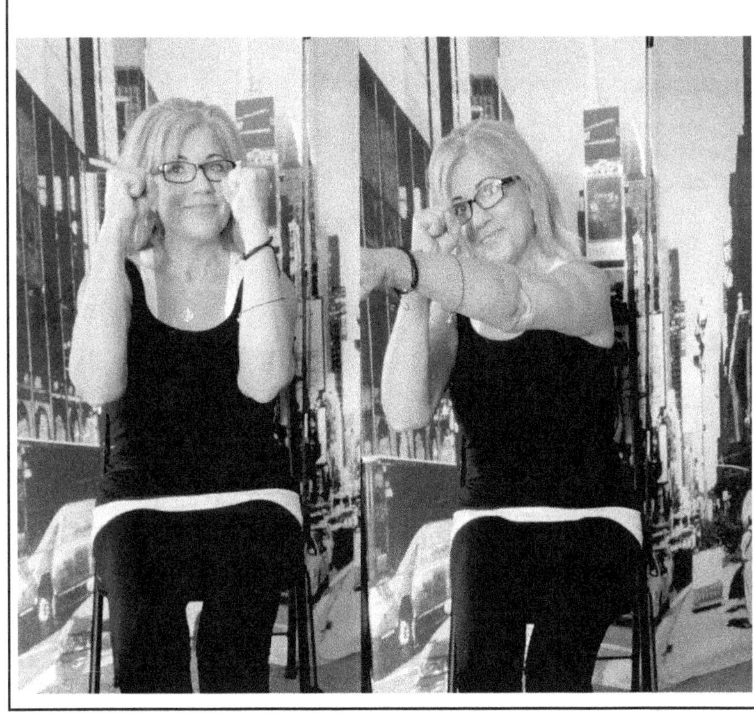

(2 of 2)

From the starting position, continue with the left arm, alternating arms with a cross body jab until you've completed 24.
(12 jabs with each arm.)

*Add some upbeat music to make this more challenging.
(and more fun too!)

Written Instructions:

Begin with your arms by your side, using a weight that is safe and comfortable for you, and okay with your doctor as well.

With palms facing out, bend your arms at the elbow, bringing the weights up to the position shown below.

Return to the starting position and repeat.
Complete a total of 12 bicep curls.

Working the Biceps

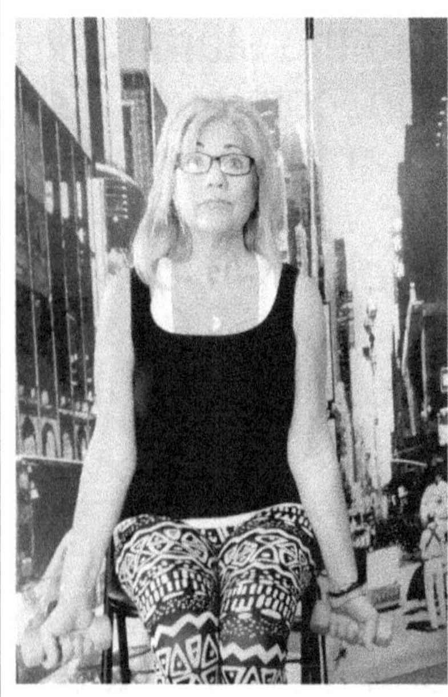 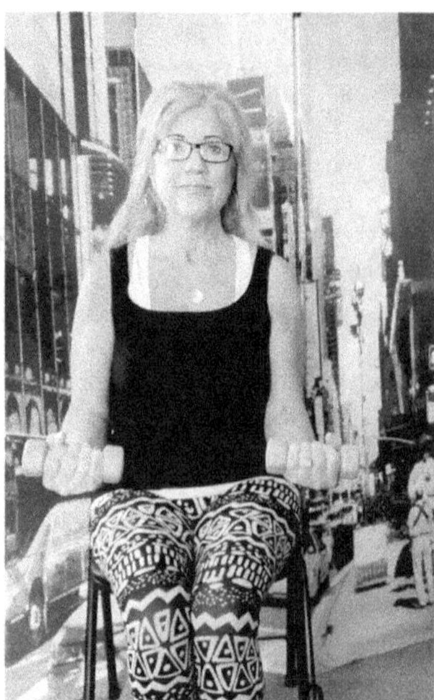 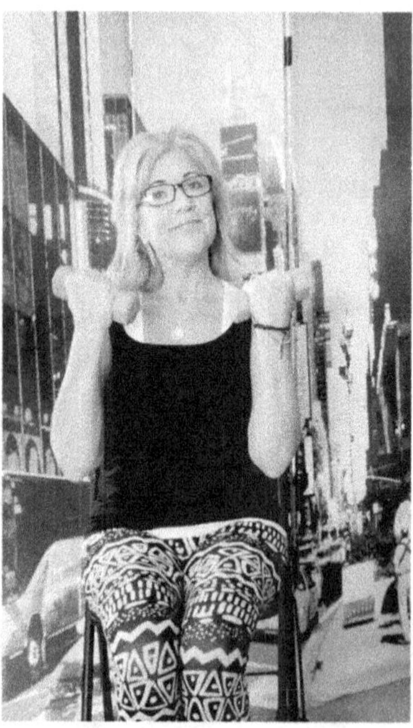

Triceps

(One arm at a time)
Begin in the starting position, with your palm facing inward, as shown.
Moving the arm from the elbow down only, extend the arm backwards as shown, until the bottom of your weight is facing the ceiling.
Return to starting position.
Complete 12 on each side.

Working the Triceps

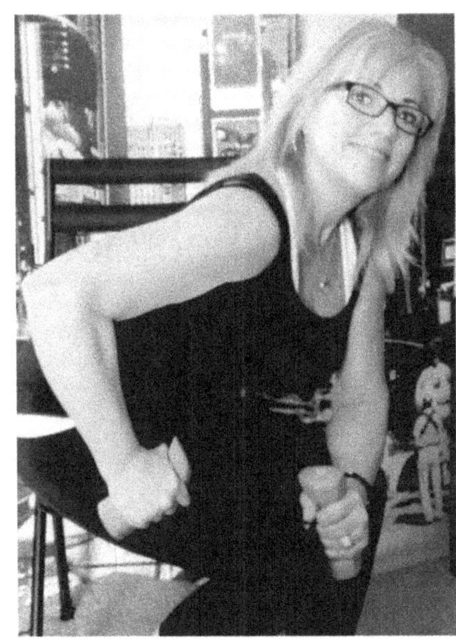
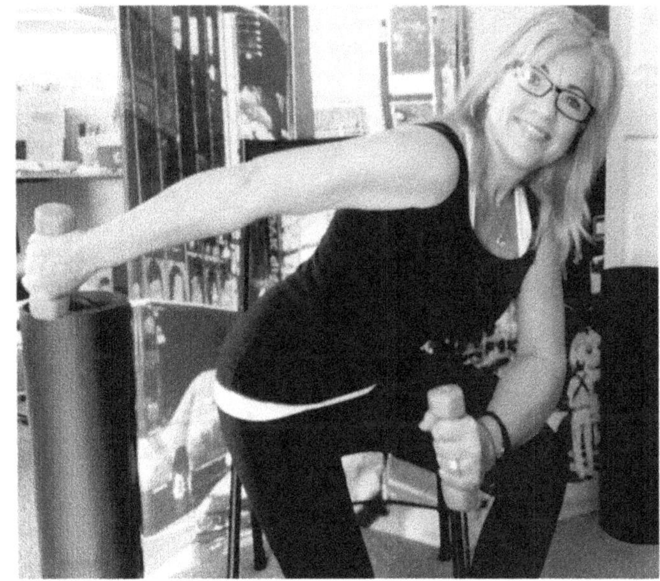

Side Stretches

In a seated position, place your feet flat on the floor,with your arms at your side and fingertips facing the floor. Begin with the right arm, (palm facing up), lift the right arm straight up, then over, until your fingertips are at 1:00. (Hold chair with opposite hand to keep balance if needed.) Return to the starting position and repeat on the other side, (11:00), for a total of 10 stretches.
(5 stretches on each side.)

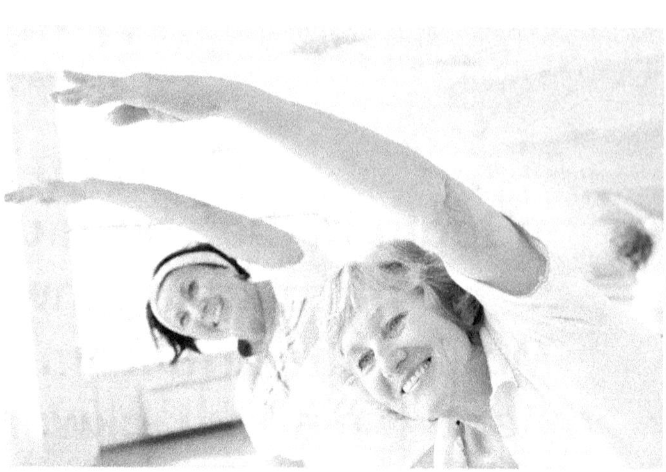

Remember to inhale in through nose and exhale through the mouth with each stretch.

Arm Stretch

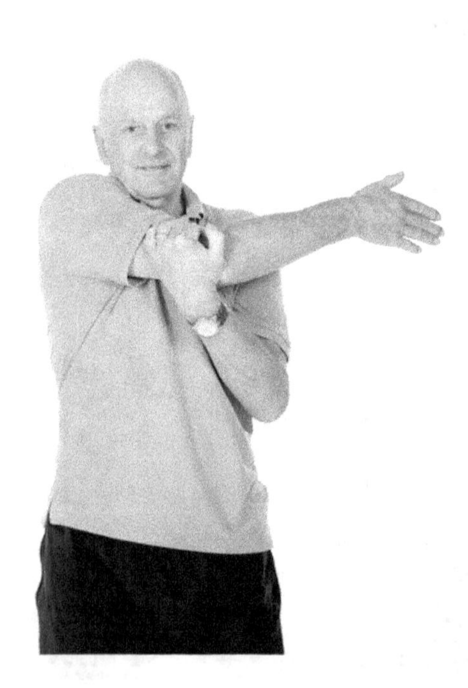

Begin with one arm straight out in front of you. Slowly move the arm across your body.
Place the opposite hand on your elbow, while gently pressing your arm in towards your body for a deeper stretch.
Hold for 10 seconds, then repeat on the opposite side.

For an optimal stretch, do your best to keep your shoulders as squared as possible.

Refer to the slide below for our final stretch

Begin with your arms down by your side, and slowly raise them until you reach the position shown.
As you are lifting your arms, take a deep breath, in through the nose. (4 seconds)
As you bring your hands back down to your side, release your breath through the mouth. (8 seconds)
(*Pursing your lips helps slow the release of breath.*)

Repeat this three times.

This is a great time to practice gratitude. Allow a few things for which you are thankful to be seen by your mind's eye as you breathe in and out.

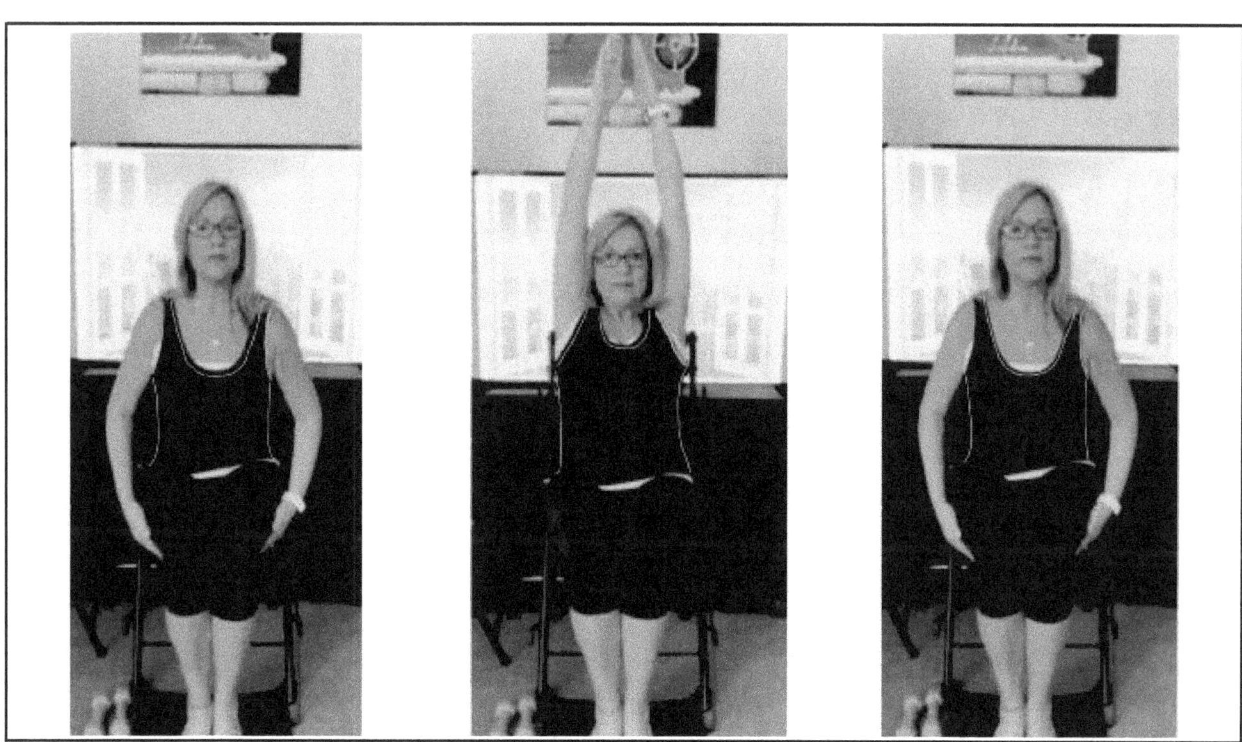

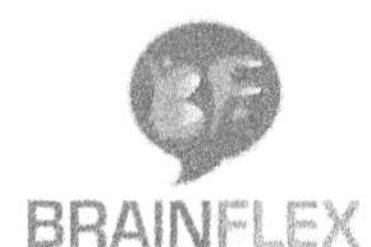

BRAINFLEX

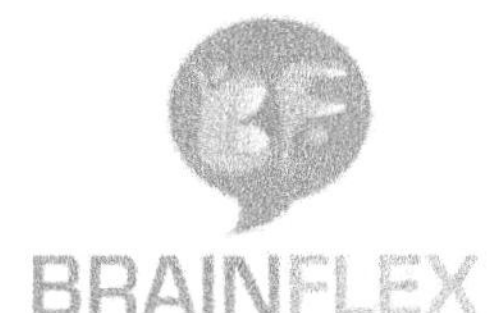

Prayer/Meditation Guide

Monthly Meditation/Prayer
Purposeful Breathing Guide
(Use w/Self-Affirmations Sheets)

Begin to play soft relaxing music. (Nature, Spa, Classical, etc.)

1. Get comfortable – Relax in a comfortable chair. Breathing in through the nose (this should take 4 seconds) then...out through the mouth, which should take about 8 seconds.
(Pursing your lips will help lengthen the time of the exhale.)
(*Repeat this breathing exercise once more.*)

2. Next, begin to relax the face muscles, (mouth, jaw), then relax the neck, shoulders, arms, hands, fingers, legs, feet, toes, and spine... letting yourself melt into the chair.

3. To begin, focus on the music while maintaining regulated breathing, [**Regulated Breathing**: *In through the nose and out through the nose, at a very steady pace, feeling the breath going in through your nose and out through your nose, noticing your belly rising and falling with each steady breath.*]

4. Next, focus on **gratitude. Thoughts of thankfulness**, allowing the people, places, things, etc., for which you are thankful to play over and over in your mind like a beautiful slide show. Focus on the word, 'Thank you'. (Hear it...say it...feel it, alongside your thoughts of gratitude.)

5. After a few minutes, focus back on the music and take two nice deep breaths (as instructed in #1), then settle back into your chair, once again, relaxing each muscle. (as instructed in #2)

BrainFlex® Wellness©

6. Choose an affirmation from your 'Self-Affirmations' sheet, and repeat the affirmation out loud, then, as you listen to the music, focus on the words you just spoke, repeating them both out loud, and in your mind, as you practice your regulated breathing and relax to the music.

7. After a few minutes, choose a second affirmation from your 'Self-Affirmation' sheet, and repeat the process again, just as you did in #6.

8. After a few more minutes, choose a third affirmation from your 'Self-Affirmation' sheet, once again, repeating the process, just as you did in #6 & #7.

9. When you feel you are ready, place your focus back on the music and take two nice deep breaths, (following the instructions in #1), then settle back into your chair, relaxing each face muscle again,(as instructed in #2). When you are finished, return to your regulated/ rhythmic breathing. (#3)

10. After a few minutes, return your focus back to gratitude and thankfulness. Once again, focusing on those things for which you are thankful...see them with your mind, as you hear the word, 'Thank You', playing over and over in your thoughts.

11. Before you finish, spend some time in prayer.

12. As you finish this time, repeat #1, taking 2-3 nice deep breaths. *(Take your time getting up. Make sure to drink plenty of water.)*

Gratitude

Take a few minutes to pause and write down some things for which you are thankful.

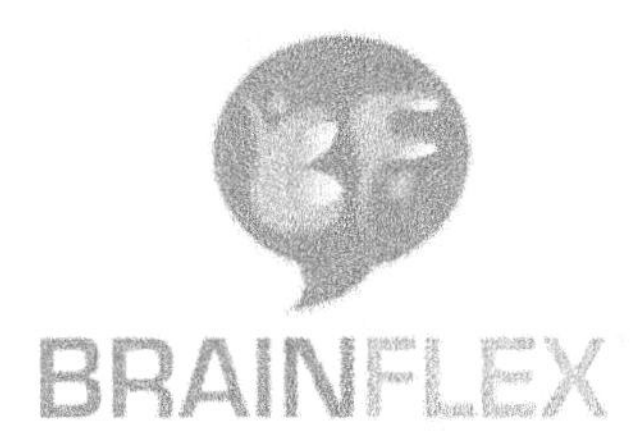

WEEK ONE

NUTRITIONAL RECIPE

Contributing to a healthier brain & body

The health benefits in the recipe's ingredients will vary with each individual and depend heavily upon each person's level of commitment to making healthy life-style choices on a consistent basis.

HEALTHY PEANUT-PRETZEL ENERGY BARS

Ingredients

1 ¼ cup of quick oats
       choose gluten free option
¼ - cup slivered almonds
½ - cup sugar free dark chocolate chips
       sweetened w/Stevia
1 ¼ cup pretzels (after crushing)
       choose gluten free option
1 - cup of all-natural peanut butter
1 - tsp vanilla
2 - TBSP ground flax seed
½ - cup of local honey

<u>Instructions</u>

1.) Line a 9 x 9 pan with parchment paper.
2.) In a separate bowl, mix all the dry ingredients.
   (oats, almonds, chocolate chips, flax seed & pretzels)
3.) Set aside portion of choc. chips & pretzels to
   sprinkle over bars after they are pressed into the pan.
4.) Add vanilla to dry ingredients and stir.
5.) In separate bowl, mix honey & natural peanut butter.
6.) Mix all ingredients together, spread into pan and press.
7.) Sprinkle remaining choc. chips & pretzels over bars.
8.) Refrigerate for one hour before slicing into squares.

<u>Oats:</u> <u>One of the healthiest grains on earth</u>

High in a very specific group of antioxidants called avenanthramides, which are solely found in oats. These have been shown to lower blood pressure levels by increasing the production of nitric oxide. This gas molecule helps dilate blood vessels & leads to better blood flow.

Manganese: 191% of RDI   **Phosphorus:** 41% of RDI
Magnesium: 34% of RDI   **Copper:** 24% of RDI
Iron: 20% of the RDI   **Vitamin B1** 39% of RDI

<u>Health Benefits: Ground Flax Seed</u>

>High in omega-3 fats, which are beneficial to
 heart and brain health
>A rich source of 'Lignans' that have been shown to
 help reduce the risk of certain cancers
>A great source of dietary fiber, which supports
 digestive health
>Helps improve cholesterol & lower blood pressure
>Contains high-quality protein, which is beneficial
     to our bones and keeps us feeling full

<u>Health Benefits: Natural Peanut Butter</u>

- High in Niacin, a nutrient that has been shown in
  research studies to help improve brain function

- High in protein, which provides energy, helps
  regulate blood sugar, and keeps the appetite
  satisfied

- The healthy fats in natural (organic) peanut butter
  are important to cardiovascular health.

- Eating foods that contain healthy fat is necessary
  for brain function.

Health Benefits: Almonds

1.) High in Magnesium, which helps the body absorb calcium
    a.) Magnesium has also been shown to help
       reduce anxiety and migraine headaches.
2.) Contains the healthy fats needed to nourish the heart & brain
3.) Loaded with antioxidants, equipping our body to fight cell
       damaging free radicals.
4.) High in vitamin E, which contributes to healthier skin
5.) High in protein, helping the body control blood sugar levels
6.) Has been shown to help control (and even lower) cholesterol
    levels

Health Benefits: Honey

- Sooths throat and helps minimize cough

- Using locally produced honey can help prevent seasonal allergies

- Contains antibacterial properties, which are beneficial to the immune system and also helps promote healthy gut bacteria

Use this space to draw, doodle, make notes, jot down a special memory, experience or an important lesson learned in life.

Brain Stimulating
Exercises
Lesson 1

<u>Reminder Page</u>

Don't forget to check off the following after you complete them today:

____ Exercise

____ Prayer/Meditation

____ Self-Affirmations

Self-Affirmations

The self-affirmations included in our workbooks are built on a healthy love of self, not an egotistical kind of love. This portion of the Aging Well program is about self-respect, knowing that you are worthy… that you are good enough…just the way you are.

It's important to say each affirmation several times out loud, even if you aren't sure you believe what you're saying. Over time, your mind's eye will begin to see the world, (this includes YOU)…in a more positive light. We believe that we're all God's creation and that it's important to Him that we love and appreciate the unique design of every person, (this includes YOU).

I am beautiful…just the way I am.

I respect myself.

I am confident in who I am.

I let go of all negative thinking.

I will replace negative thoughts with positive ones.

LESSON 1: Research & Discussion: Right Brain vs Left Brain

The left side of the brain is primarily where we process logic, sequence, rational and analytical thinking, (and solve most math problems). The right side of the brain plays a very important role in our personality and basically in how we behave in general. However, for some, the left brain may have the tendency to try and push the right brain aside and take control.

One way in which our right brain is helpful, is in the area of subjective thinking. Our right brain is where we experience intuition, which influences subjective thinking.

"I like that dress." or "Those flowers are beautiful". *These are subjective because they are 'opinions', not facts.*

Our left brain is helpful in the area of objective thinking, when it is required that we pay attention to facts, rather than 'feelings'.

"The sun is hot." or "The earth is round."
These are objective statements because they have been proven to be true.

Both the left and right sides of the brain are necessary, especially for learning & relearning. However, generally speaking, most of the education we experienced during our 'formative' years focused on teaching the facts.

(These subjects include language, science, math, and history, which primarily use the left hemisphere of the brain.) *The brain always uses both hemispheres, each with certain responsibilities.*

It's usually not until later in life that we are exposed to philosophy, psychology, and other subjects that require more 'free thinking' and subjective input.

The good news is…it's never too late to increase our use of both hemispheres of the brain, which is what we do in each BrainFlex Workbook.

A few ways you can exercise the 'right brain':

- o Expressing visually through art and poetry
- o Drawing
- o Writing
- o Skits/Role play
- o Games that involve 'word play'
- o Listening to the symphony
- o Cooking
- o Writing stories

MATH SKILLS REVIEW

Since math is a skill we use often, it's very important to practice on a regular basis.

951	661	742	321	769
549	573	759	641	560
423	144	255	714	911
+ 699	+ 373	+ 161	+ 429	+ 152

33	32	41	94	25
18	17	14	15	28
17	21	33	81	15
20	90	80	28	46
65	99	23	89	94
+ 10	+ 69	+ 67	+ 19	+ 68

$5.00	$7.00	$1.50	$8.50	$8.50
+ $9.50	+ $8.00	+ $3.00	+ $9.00	+ $5.00

$9)\overline{95}$ $3)\overline{88}$ $2)\overline{80}$ $7)\overline{77}$ $7)\overline{45}$

$4)\overline{236}$ $5)\overline{165}$ $7)\overline{518}$ $6)\overline{516}$ $8)\overline{448}$

Month: June

SUN.	MON.	TUES.	WED.	THURS.	FRI.	SAT
		1	2	3	4	5
6	7	8	9	10	11	12
13	14	15	16	17	18	19
20	21	22	23	24	25	26
27	28	29	30	31		

Refer to the calendar above to answer the following questions.

1.) Becky has invited her friends to her wedding in Hawaii, which will take place on June 19th. They sent their invitations out via email, which means everyone received their invite on the same day. Although everyone was excited, they all wished they didn't have to wait another week and 5 days to attend the wedding. On what day and date did everyone receive their invitation? ______________ ______________ *(On the calendar above, place the letter 'W' on the day the guests received their invitation.)*

2.) Kem had an appointment for a massage on June 3rd. However, just a few minutes before she was to leave, the salon called to inform her that the appointment would need to be changed. Her new appointment is two weeks and four days from her original appointment. On what day and date is her new appointment? ______________ __________
(On the calender above, place the letter 'K' on her new appointment date.)

3.) Stacey runs a busy hair salon in the heart of downtown Dayton, Ohio. She recently noticed that she had overbooked herself on June 5th and 12th. She has decided to move four appointments scheduled on these days. Mel's appointment for June 5th has been moved two weeks out. Jim was scheduled on the same day, and his appointment has been moved one week and two days out. Mitch and Dan were both scheduled on June 12th; Mitch's appointment has been moved out one week and four days, while Dan's was only moved three days out. On the calendar above, write the names of each client on the new days/dates they have been scheduled.

Exercise: Language & Vocabulary
Write either an antonym or a synonym for each word listed below.

1. Antonym for **awareness** _______________________

2. Synonym for **confusion** _______________________

3. Antonym for **soothed** _______________________

4. Synonym for **frightened** _______________________

5. Antonym for **excited** _______________________

6. Synonym for **sad** _______________________

7. Antonym for **joyfulness** _______________________

8. Synonym for **suffering** _______________________

9. Antonym for **underwhelmed** _______________________

10. Synonym for **flooded** _______________________

11. Antonym for **calm** _______________________

12. Synonym for **astonished** _______________________

13. Antonym for **ordinary** _______________________

14. Synonym for **honored** _______________________

15. Antonym for **shy** _______________________

Kevin recently retired, and each night when he goes to bed, he wonders where his time went that day and what he accomplished. We're going to help him track his time by using the clocks on the next page to answer the following questions.

1. On clock #1, draw in the hands to show the time as 5:15, which will indicate the time Kevin gets up each morning.

2. Three hours and fifteen minutes later, Kevin finds himself in front of the television to catch up on the morning news. On clock #2, draw in the hands to show the time Kevin turns on the morning news.

3. Two hours and 10 minutes later, the doorbell rings. The postman has delivered a package for which Kevin has been waiting on for quite some time. *(Kevin is a frequent shopper on QVC.)* On clock #3, draw in the hands to show the time the package was delivered.

4. One hour and 40 minutes later, Kevin opened the package, pulled out the tip and the windings, but couldn't find the guide or the hook keeper.
On clock #4 draw in the hands to show when he opened the package.

5. Thirty-five minutes later, Kevin finally found the guide and the hook keeper in the trash, after realizing that he had thrown out a portion of the box with the missing parts still in it. On clock #5, draw in the hands to show the time he found the items.

6. Two hours and 25 minutes later, Kevin had put his item together and was ready to try it out. On clock #6, draw in the hands to show the current time.

7. One hour and fifty-five minutes later, Kevin returned from the lake, and had brought dinner back with him. On clock #7, draw in the hands to show the time Kevin returned from the lake.

8. His wife, Sheri explained that supper was already started, and it would be ready in 30 minutes. On clock #8, draw the hands to show 'dinner time'.

9. Kevin went to bed at 9pm each night. After finishing dinner, he looked at the clock and couldn't believe he only had two hours and 15 minutes before bed. On clock #9, draw the hands to show what time Kevin finished dinner.

BONUS: What was the item Kevin received in the mail? _______________________

BrainFlex® Wellness©

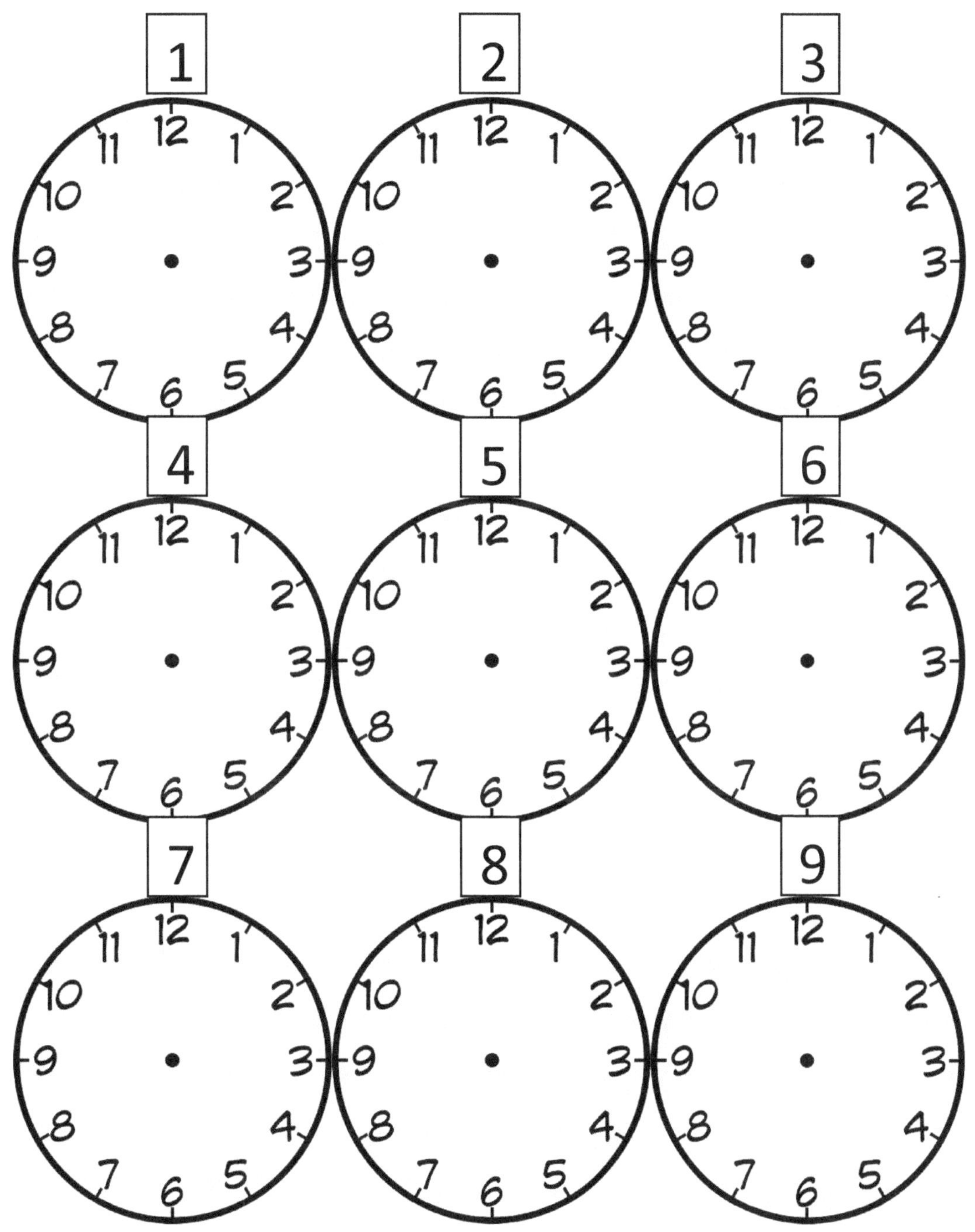

Use the clocks above and follow the instructions on the previous page to exercise your time orientation and math skills.

Use this space for doodling, taking notes,
or just to jot down a special thought or memory.

50

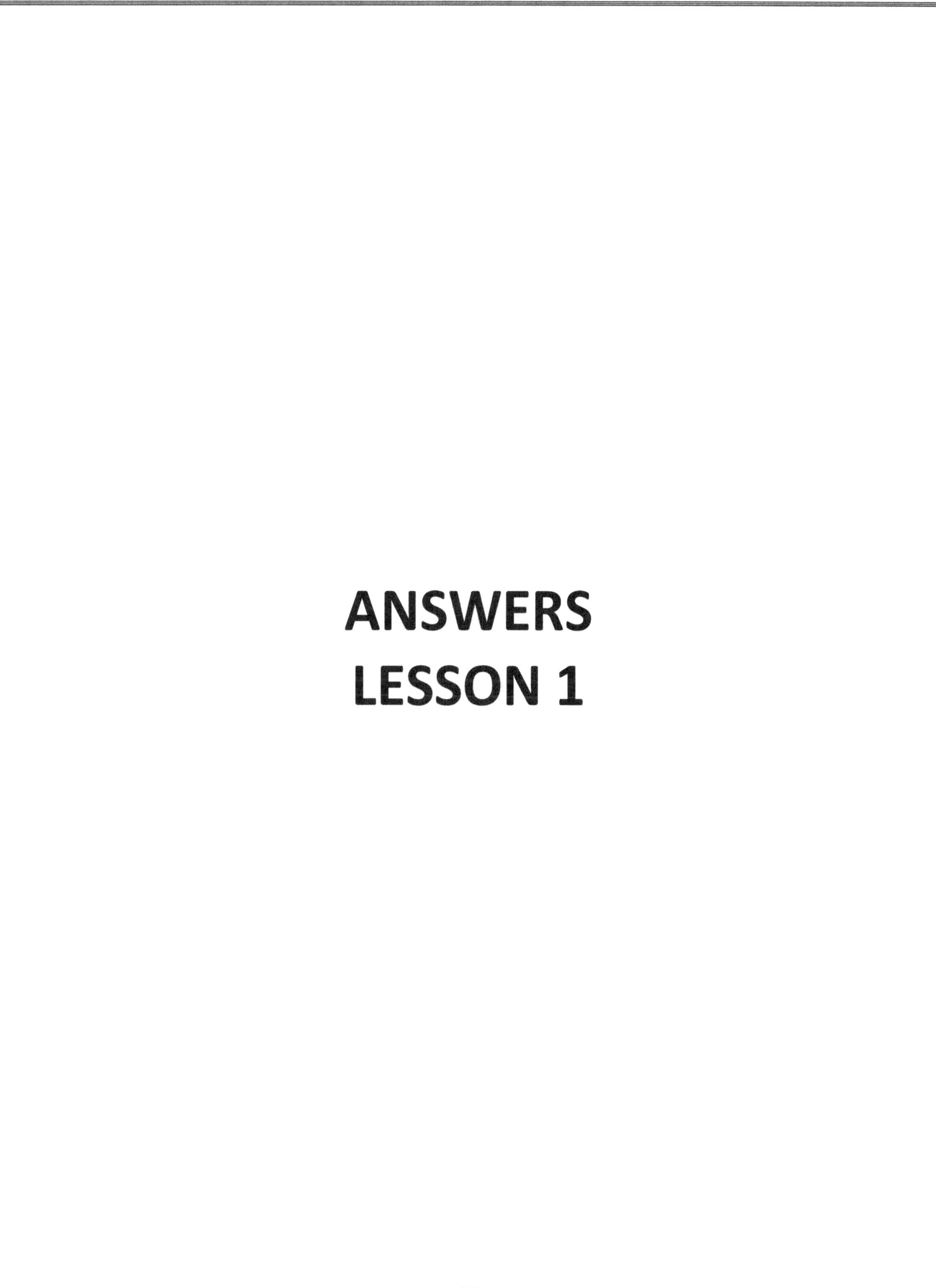

ANSWERS
LESSON 1

ANSWERS TO LESSON 1

Answers Math Skills Review

Addition

2622	1751	1917	2105	2392

Addition

163	328	258	326	276

Adding Money

$14.50	$15.00	$4.50	$17.50	$13.50

Division

10 r-5	29 r-1	40	11	6 r-3
59	33	74	86	56

Answers to 'Calendar-Time Orientation-Attention to Detail

1.Becky has invited her friends to her wedding in Hawaii, which will take place on June 19th. They sent their invitations out via email, which means everyone received their invite on the same day. Although everyone was excited, they all wished they didn't have to wait another week and 5 days to attend the wedding. What day and date did everyone receive their invitation? **12 days before June 19th is Monday, June 7th. (7 days in one week + 5 days = 12 days)**

2.If Kem's appointment was on the 3rd, and it was rescheduled for two weeks and four days from the 3rd, then her appointment would be on **Monday, JUNE 21st. (Two weeks = 14 days + 4 days = 18 days) (18 + 3 = 21)**

3.Stacey moved Mel two weeks out from June 5th, making her new appointment on **June 19th (14 days after June 5th).** Jim was moved one week and two days out from June 5th, making his new appointment on **June 14th (9 days after June 5th).** Mitch was moved from the 12th to **June 23rd. (11 days after June 12th).** Dan was moved to **June 15th, 3 days after his June 12th appointment.**

SUN.	MON.	TUES.	WED.	THURS.	FRI.	SAT
		1	2	3	4	5
6	W 7	8	9	10	11	12
13	Jim 14	Dan 15	16	17	18	Mel 19
20	K 21	22	Mitch 23	24	25	26
27	28	29	30	31		

ANSWERS TO LESSON 1

Answers to-Exercise: Language & Vocabulary
(answers may vary)

1. Antonym for **awareness** - ALOOF

2. Synonym for **confusion** - CHAOS

3. Antonym for **soothed** – IRRITATED

4. Synonym for **frightened** - SCARED

5. Antonym for **excited** - INDIFFERENT

6. Synonym for **sad** – MELANCHOLY

7. Antonym for **joyfulness** - SADNESS

8. Synonym for **suffering** - MISERY

9. Antonym for **underwhelmed** - OVERWHELMED

10. Synonym for **flooded** – INUNDATED

11. Antonym for **calm** - ANXIOUS

12. Synonym for **astonished** - SHOCKED

13. Antonym for **ordinary** – DISTINGUISHED

14. Synonym for **honored** - RESPECTED

15. Antonym for **shy** - OUTGOING

Answers-Maintain CLOCK-TIME ORIENTATION

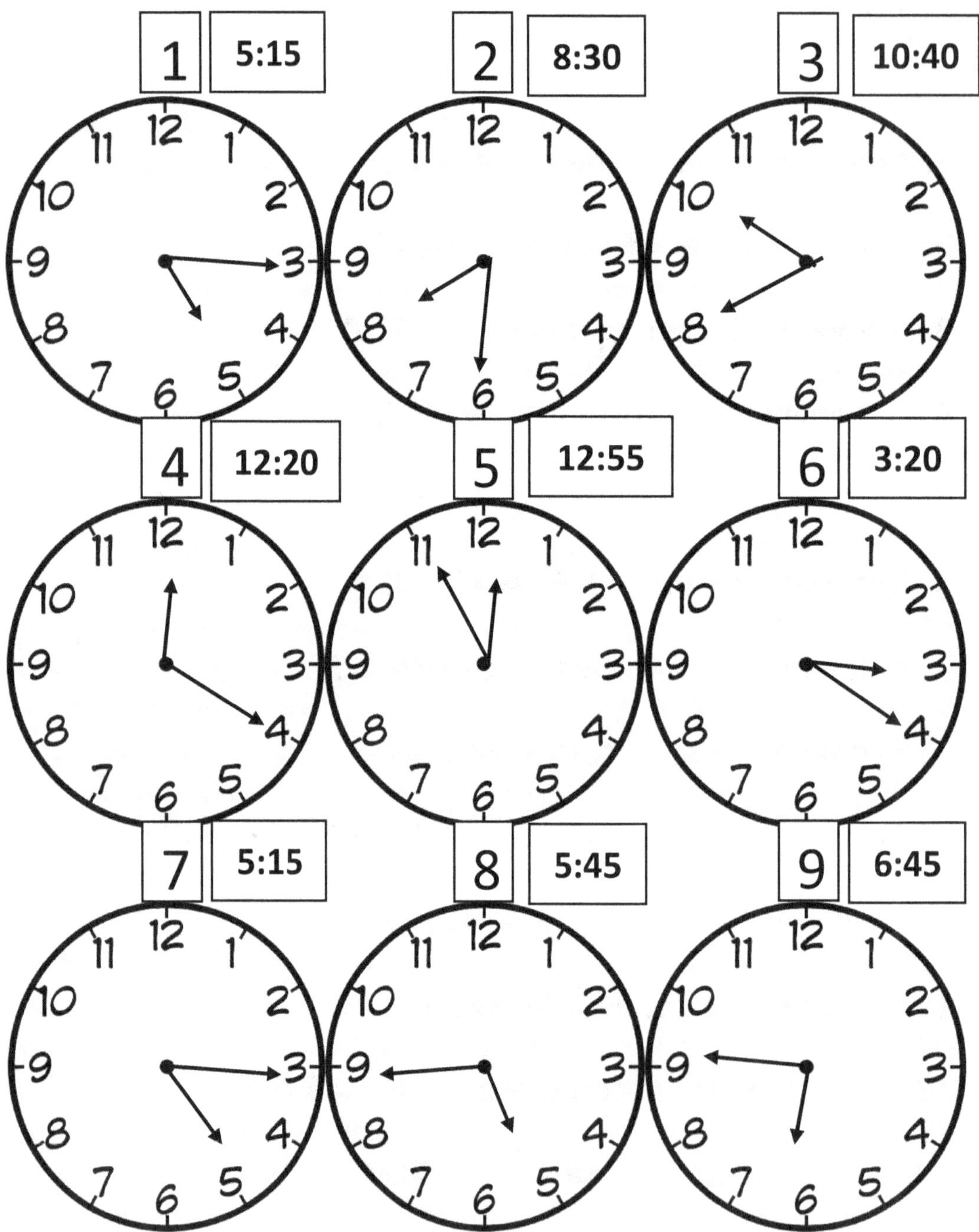

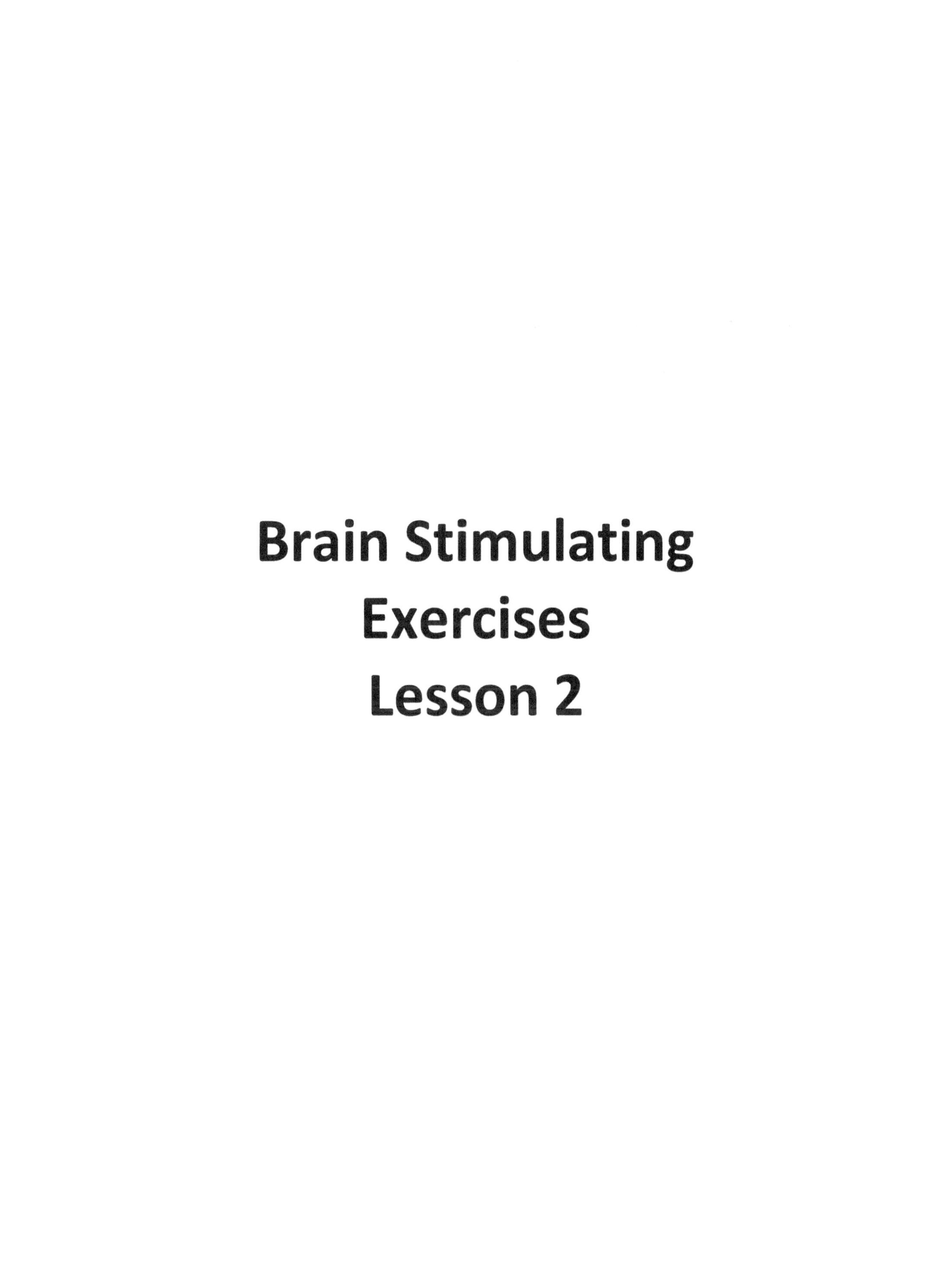

Brain Stimulating
Exercises
Lesson 2

<u>Reminder Page</u>

Don't forget to check off the following after you complete them today:

_____ **Exercise**

_____ **Prayer/Meditation**

_____ **Self-Affirmations**

Self-Affirmations

I have a strong body and a healthy brain.

I free myself of all bitterness and unforgiveness.

I can see my true beauty…within and without.

I choose to assume and believe the best about others.

I choose to believe what God says about me.

I am loved and accepted by those I love.

<u>LESSON 2: Research-Discussion Sheet: Exercising for Brain Plasticity</u>

>One thing we say repeatedly is that age doesn't matter when it comes to learning. Although, as we age, it may take us a little longer to learn something new, we can still continue learning throughout our lifetime.
(Repetition is key!)

>Many researchers across the globe also agree that we can continue learn as we age, which is what the term 'Brain Plasticity' means.
(We can grow new neural pathways as long as we are committed to doing so.)

>Researchers agree that we need make a concerted effort and remain committed to all the components important to brain health if we want to experience the best outcomes from life-long learning.

These components are: Exercise, Healthy Diet, Brain Stimulation, and Social Connections. (*In addition, we now understand the impact that healthy sleep patterns and a positive mindset have on the aging brain.*)

Although each of these important components are required to 'age well', for the purpose of this research and discussion sheet, we will focus on Exercise.

<u>Exercise</u> is an area of research where the positive impact on brain health is undeniable.

->Exercise improves the flow of oxygen throughout our body, which in turn, benefits both the body and the brain, including memory.

->Exercise has been shown in repeated studies to provide our brains with *'fight'*, some researchers describe this fight as ***'reverse aging'***.

->Exercise creates an overall feeling of well-being through the release of 'feel good' chemicals. (neurotransmitters)

->Exercise increases the number of dendrites in the brain. Dendrites are extensions of our nerve cells. Their job is to receive electrical impulses from other cells and then communicate those messages to other parts of the brain.

References

Smale, T. (2017, December 12). *8 Ways to Improve Your Brain Power*. Retrieved from Entrepreneur:

https://www.entrepreneur.com/article/250417

MATH SKILLS REVIEW

$$8\overline{)720} \qquad 8\overline{)304} \qquad 9\overline{)774} \qquad 3\overline{)162} \qquad 5\overline{)285}$$

$3.50	$3.50	$1.50	$1.50	$0.50
$7.50	$0.50	$9.50	$3.00	$8.50
+ $4.50	+ $9.00	+ $7.50	+ $9.00	+ $3.00

929	933	579	169	169
898	469	332	654	490
282	976	272	861	231
+ 902	+ 690	+ 519	+ 389	+ 572

$$4\overline{)236} \qquad 5\overline{)165} \qquad 7\overline{)518} \qquad 6\overline{)516} \qquad 8\overline{)448}$$

1. Sue's best friend, Jill, recently stole her boyfriend, and one evening, while walking through the park, she unexpectedly ran into them. Pretending not to see them, she walked in the opposite direction, but was shocked when she heard Jill yell across the park, "Hey, all is fair in _______ _____ ______."

2. Marge was frustrated when she saw the stock market results that day. For weeks, she had planned on purchasing stock in *RTN Tech*, but kept putting it off, and today their stock skyrocketed. She sat at her desk, with her head resting in her hands and sighed, "When will I learn that time and tide _______ _____ _________?"

3. While staying with his grandparents, Austin decided to go out with a friend. He knew they would not approve of this particular person. He could already hear his grandpa saying, "It only takes one bad ________ ____
______ ____ ________ _________."

4. Jan opened the door and was speechless when she saw her first-grade teacher, Ms. Sawyer, standing there! "Well hello Jan, I haven't seen you since you were…knee high _____ ____ __________."

5. Angela is heartbroken over the recent break-up with her fiancé, so she made the decision to move. She's clinging to the ole cliche'… "out of __________ out of ________."

6. Anna had found the man of her dreams, but thankfully her father was a police officer and decided to do a little investigating, which only confirmed his suspicion. After dinner one night, he sat Anna down and said, "Honey… he's as slippery as ___ _______."

7. Maria was 16 and excited to start her new job. Only a few weeks after starting, she purchased a brand new car. Unfortunately, six weeks into flipping hamburgers, she began to hate her job, but she had just purchased a new car, so now she had a large car payment to make. She asked her father if she could quit her job, assuring him that she could easily find another job. Her father paused, then put his hand on hers and said, "Honey, I know things seem hard, but…when the going gets tough _____ ________ ______
________". After another long pause, he added, "Always remember…
"A bird in the hand is worth more than ______ ____ ______ _________."

Practice your comprehension and recall by answering the questions related to the seven scenarios on the previous page.
Try your best not to refer back to the sceneries if possible.

1. What was the name of Sue's best friend? _______________________

2. What was the name of the stock in which Marge wished she had invested? _______________________

3. What was Austin planning on doing even though he knew his grandparents would not approve? _______________________

____

4. What was the name of Jan's first grade teacher who shocked her with a surprise visit? _______________________

5. Why did Angela decide to move away? _______________________

6. Anna thought she had found the man of her dreams, but fortunately, her father was a ___________ ___________, and did some checking on him.

7. What was Maria's job that she hated so much? _______________________

____

Below, write five (5) cliché's that you recall using frequently.

1) ____

____

2) ____

____

3) ____

____

4) ____

____

5) ____

____

BrainFlex® Wellness©

Warm Up Exercise: Assigning Value ~ Visual Orientation

Pictured below are six different bricks, each with different weight values, in pounds. Use these bricks as a guide to answer the questions.

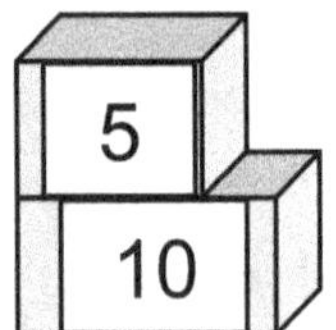
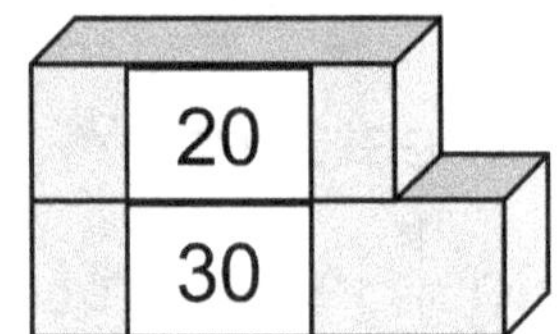
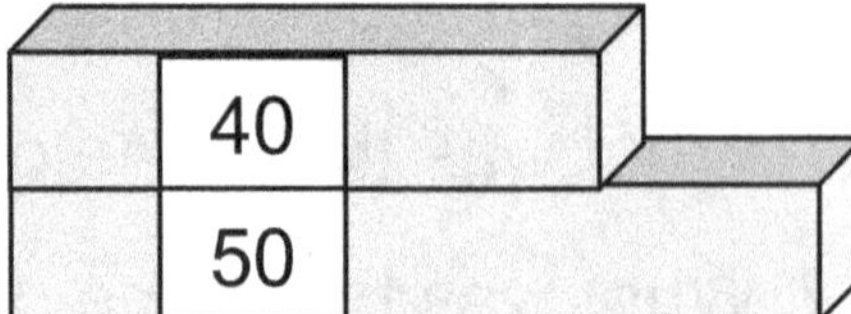

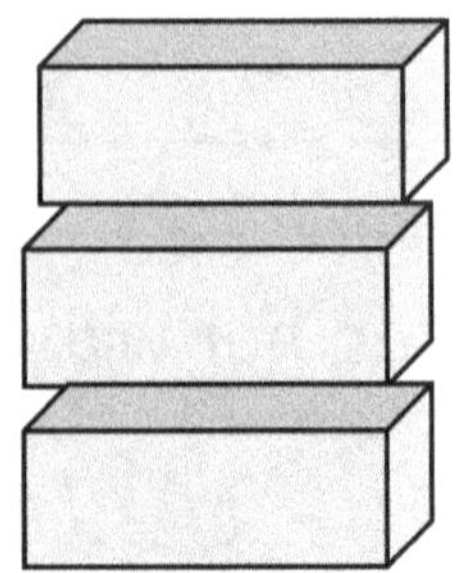

1. According to the examples above, how much would this stack of bricks weigh if the actual weight was 3 times the weight shown on each brick? _______

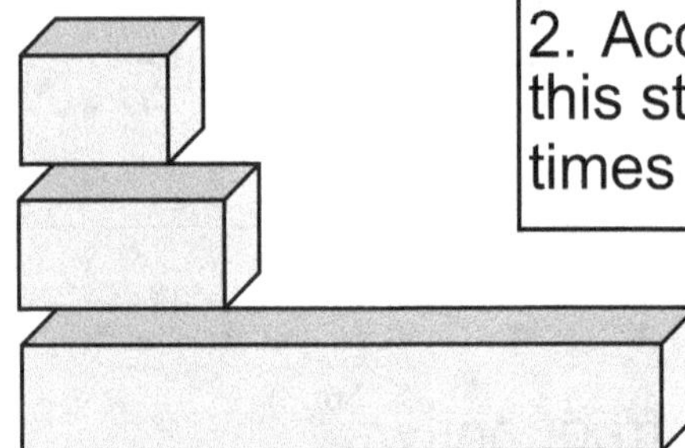

2. According to the examples above, how much would this stack of bricks weigh if the actual weight was 6 times the weight shown on each brick? _______

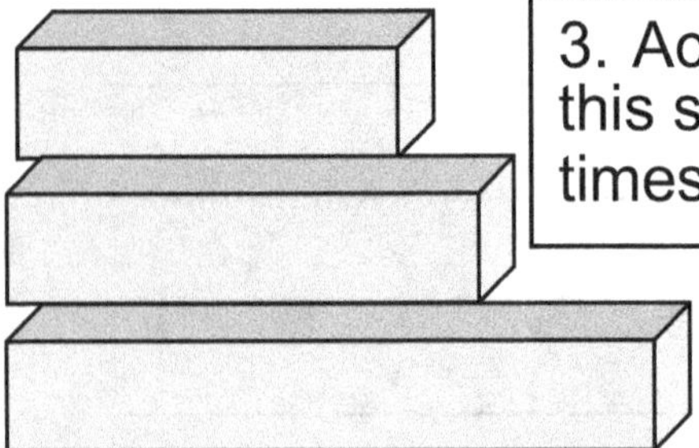

3. According to the examples above, how much would this stack of bricks weigh if the actual weight was 8 times the weight shown on each brick? _______

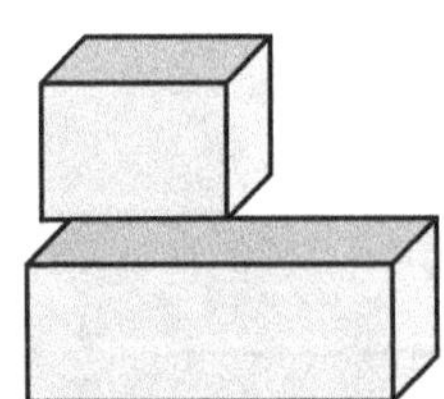

4. According to the examples above, how much would this stack of bricks weigh if the actual weight was 10 times the weight shown on each brick? _______

REFLECTION

Take a few minutes to pause and think about the past week.
Write about two or three special moments you would like to
relive and why you feel this way.

____

____

____

____

____

____

____

____

____

____

____

____

____

Use this space for doodling, taking notes,
or just to jot down a special thought or memory.

64

ANSWERS
LESSON 2

Answers to Math Skills Review

90	38	86	54	57
$15.50	$13.00	$18.50	$13.50	$12.00
3011	3068	1702	2073	1462
59	33	74	86	56

Answers-Exercising Long-Term Memory w/Story & Comprehension w/ Recall PG 1 of 2

1. All is fair in love and war.
2. Time and tide wait for no one.
3. It only takes one...**bad apple to spoil the whole barrel.**
4. Knee high to a grasshopper.
5. Out of sight, out of mind.
6. He's as slippery as an eel.
7. When the going gets tough, the tough get going. A bird in the hand is worth two in the bush.

Answers-Exercising Long-Term Memory w/Story & Comprehension w/ Recall PG 2 of 2

1. Jill
2. RTN Tech
3. He was going out with someone he knew his grandparents would not approve of.
4. Ms. Sawyer
5. She was heartbroken over the recent break-up with her fiancé.
6. Police Officer
7. Flipping burgers

Answers: Name Five Cliché's

Answers to this portion of the exercise will vary according to individual.

Answers to Warm up Exercise: Assigning Value~Visual Orientation

1. **180** (20+20+20) = 60 (60x3=180)
2. **390** (5+10+50)=65 (65x6=390)
3. **960** (30+40+50) =120 (120x8)=960
4. **250** (5+20) =25 (25x10)=250

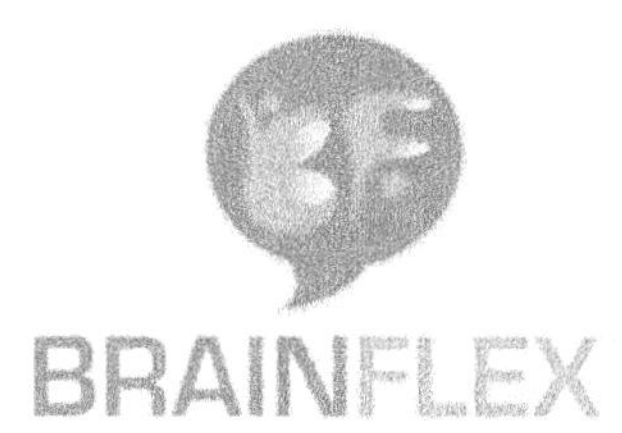

WEEK TWO

NUTRITIONAL RECIPE

Contributing to a healthier brain & body

The health benefits in the recipe's ingredients will vary with each individual and depend heavily upon each person's level of commitment to making healthy life-style choices on a consistent basis.

Avocado Tomato Salad

Ingredients

2 avocados

8 oz. grape tomatoes

1 large cucumber

1 cup garbanzo beans

1/3 cup red onion

1/3 cup cilantro

1 lime, juiced

Salt to taste

Instructions—Part One (1)

- Dice cucumber, place in a large mixing bowl.

- Half or quarter tomatoes, add to bowl.

- Finely dice red onion, add to bowl.

Instructions—Part Two (2)

- Roughly chop cilantro, removing stems.
  Add to mixing bowl.

- Rinse and drain garbanzo beans.
  Add 1 cup to bowl.

- Peel avocados and remove pits.
  Dice into chunks.

Instructions—Part Three (3)

- ▶ Add lime juice and salt to the bowl and stir.

- ▶ Let sit for about 20 minutes before eating
  This allows the flavors time to blend.

- ▶ Best enjoyed within 1-2 days.

Health Benefits:

Avocados...

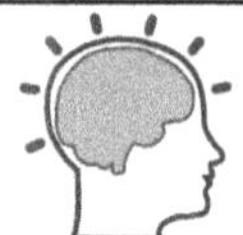

- ▶ Are high in brain-healthy fats
  An amazing brain healthy food!

- ▶ Can help reduce inflammation

- ▶ Have been shown to reduce cholesterol and contribute to heart health

- ▶ Are high in potassium, a necessary mineral that supports kidney health

Health Benefits:

Tomatoes...

- Are very high in anti-oxidants

- Contribute to a healthier immune system

- Have been shown to decrease the risk of some types of cancers

- Support cardiovascular health

- Contain folic acid, which can help reduce symptoms of depression

Health Benefits:

Garbanzo Beans...

➢ Include a particular carbohydrate that helps control blood sugar levels

➢ Are high in the protein necessary to maintain muscle

➢ Like other legumes, these beans are made of complex carbohydrates that are digested slowly, then used by the body for energy.

Use this space to jot down an important
lesson life has taught you.

Brain Stimulating
Exercises
Lesson 3

<u>Reminder Page</u>

74

Don't forget to check off the following after you complete them today:

_____ **Exercise**

_____ **Prayer/Meditation**

_____ **Self-Affirmations**

<u>SELF AFFIRMATIONS</u>

I AM CAPABLE AND STRONG.

MY CONFIDENCE IS INCREASING.

GOD WILL STRENGTHEN ME TO DO THE THINGS I NEED TO DO.

I AM PROTECTED FROM THE NEGATIVE WORDS OF OTHERS.

NO ONE DECIDES MY VALUE AND WORTH.

LESSON 3: Research-Discussion Sheet: Why Brain Training is So Important?

1. Research shows that we can radically improve our chances of maintaining a fit brain when we participate in activities that challenge the brain. It's important to engage in these types of activities daily if we want to experience the best outcomes.

2. Participating in brain stimulating activities can enhance your ability to process information and strengthen your reasoning skills.

3. When you participate in these activities, your brain receives the following benefits:

   a. Your neurons are stimulated, causing them to be more active, which in turn, allows the neurons to receive more oxygen and other nutritional elements.

   b. The stimulation that takes place in the brain during challenging activities boosts the connections between synapses.

   c. Since our neurons are kept active during these activities, they are able to produce even more neurons.

   d. While engaging in the activities in this workbook, your neurons are nurtured, which researchers say, will help them to last longer.

4. You've often heard the phrase, 'use it or lose it'. This phrase can be applied to the muscles in our body as well as to the neural pathways in our brain. This is why it's so important to stay committed to engaging in activities every day.

5. Of course, we know how a brain healthy diet and regular exercise contributes to our overall physical fitness, but it also provides a tremendous benefit to our mental fitness as well. In order for us to experience these benefits, a commitment to a healthy lifestyle should be a priority.

Remember: *Happy and Healthy is an outfit that looks good on everyone!*

References

Glasshouse, N. (2018, June 10). *Why Brain Training is Important*. Retrieved from Conscious Float:
        https://consciousfloat.com/why-brain-training-is-important/

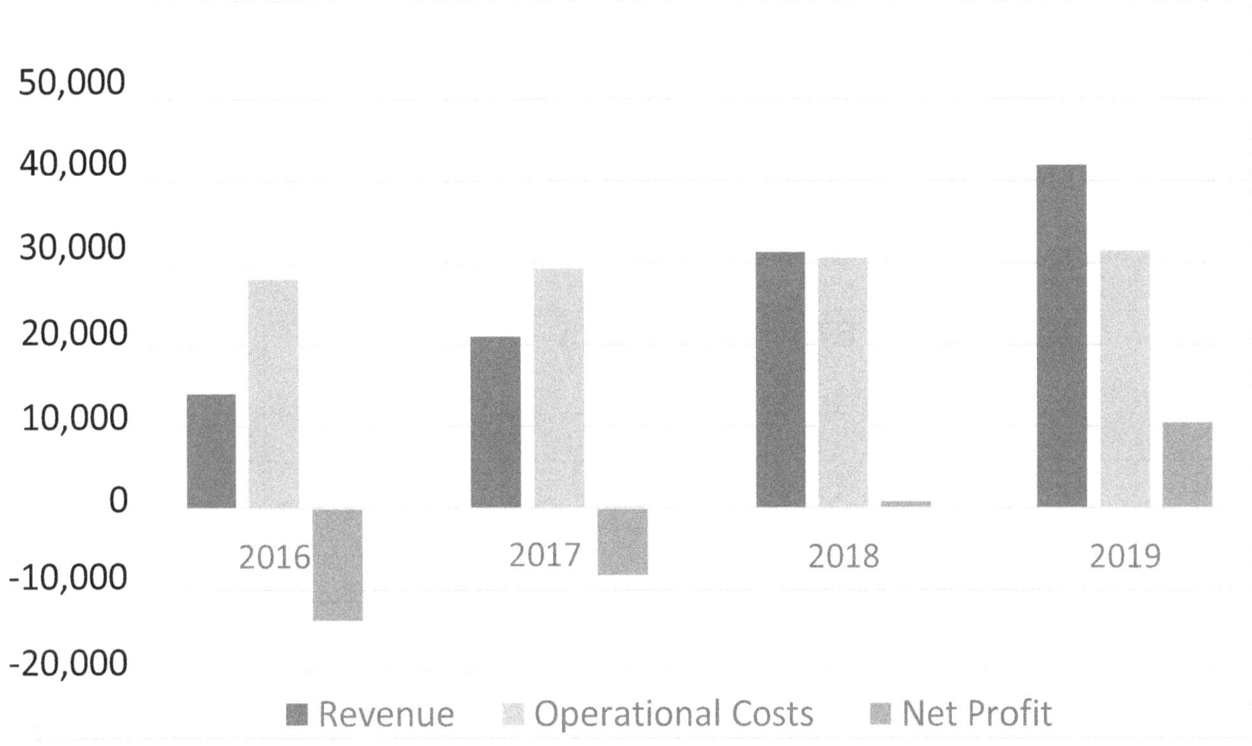

The above graph shows the last four years of revenue, operating cost, and net profit of a small business, called "Read Already", which is a unique and eclectic bookstore that primarily sells gently used books. In 2016, however, they began selling new books and magazines as well.

Use the graph to answer the following questions.

1.) In which year did the bookstore finally earn a profit and how much was the approximate amount of profit earned? _________ $ _________

2.) In which year did the bookstore experience its greatest loss and how much was the approximate amount of the loss? _________ $_________

3.) In which year did the bookstore earn the most revenue and approximately, how much revenue was earned? _________ $_________

The chart below represents the revenue, operational cost and net profit/loss for an auto repair company. Determine the net loss and/or profit for each year.

Year	Revenue	Operational Costs	"Net Profit/Loss"
2016	14,800	28,000	(loss)
2017	21,000	29,400	(loss)
2018	31,300	30,600	(profit)
2019	42,000	31,500	(profit)

Logic-Sequence
Determine the Pattern & Finish the Sequence

10,000	1,000	100	10	100	1000			
750	725	700	675	650	625			
20	22	26	32	40	50			
15	30	60	120	240	480			

LOGICAL and ILLOGICAL RIDDLES:

1.) People hire me to kill, and everyone knows it's me. However, I am neither in jail, nor am I free? What am I?

I am an E __ __ E __ M __ __ __ T __ R

(Hint: Call someone to help, there are ants in my kitchen again!)

2.) A man was born in 1955, how is it that today is his 18th birthday?
Explain: He was _______ in _______ _______
(Hint: Where 'exactly' would you visit a baby on their actual birthday?)

3.) I can travel from here to there by disappearing, and from there to here by reappearing. **I am the __ __ __ __ __ __ '__'**
(Hint: It's simply a matter of spelling)

4.) A man in Florida recently legally married three women, one was from Las Vegas, one lived in California and the other in Miami. **How was this legal? He was ___________________**
(Hint: 'Dearly beloved, we are gathered here today.')

Riddles-Overall Brain Challenge/Thought Process Exercise

1. What promise did Eve make to Adam after they were removed from the Garden of Eden?
Eve promised to turn over __   N __ __   __ __ __ F

2. What do you call a duck that hangs out with ducks that are smarter than he? A   W___ ___ ____   Q ___ ___ ___ ___ ___ ___

3. Why do some birds fly south in the winter?
Because it's too __ __ R   __ __   __ A __ __.

4. What's the best way to keep a skunk from smelling?
Put a C __ __ __ __ __ __ - P __ __ on his __ __ S __.

5. What do people call a man who is constantly wiring for money? An E ___ ___ ___ T ___ ___ C ___ ___ N

6. Where were English kings typically crowned?
___ N T H ___ ___ ___   ___ ___ ___ ___ S

7. How would you recognize a happy motorcyclist?
By the number of ___ ___ G ___ in his T ___ ___ ___ ___

8. What kind of pill would take you to the moon?
A space ___ ___ P ___ ___ ___ ___

9. Backwards I am heavy, forwards I am NOT. What am I?
A ___ ___ ___

10. Determine a synonym for each of the follow three words and you'll have a well known cliche'. 'unhappy adores visitors'
M___ ___ ___ ___ ___   L___ ___ ___ ___   C___ ___ ___ ___ ___ ___

Foundation Skills Review

$$6)\overline{312} \qquad 8)\overline{544} \qquad 5)\overline{50} \qquad 7)\overline{427} \qquad 4)\overline{108}$$

$$3)\overline{35} \qquad 4)\overline{72} \qquad 7)\overline{26} \qquad 1)\overline{94} \qquad 5)\overline{20}$$

45	14	14	98	51
23	79	19	82	97
66	86	56	91	98
39	67	13	75	35
21	25	56	97	59
+ 57	+ 81	+ 58	+ 33	+ 96

86	28	75	16	14
51	97	52	41	28
37	52	73	37	12
14	71	49	35	24
88	61	78	96	84
+ 95	+ 11	+ 66	+ 80	+ 78

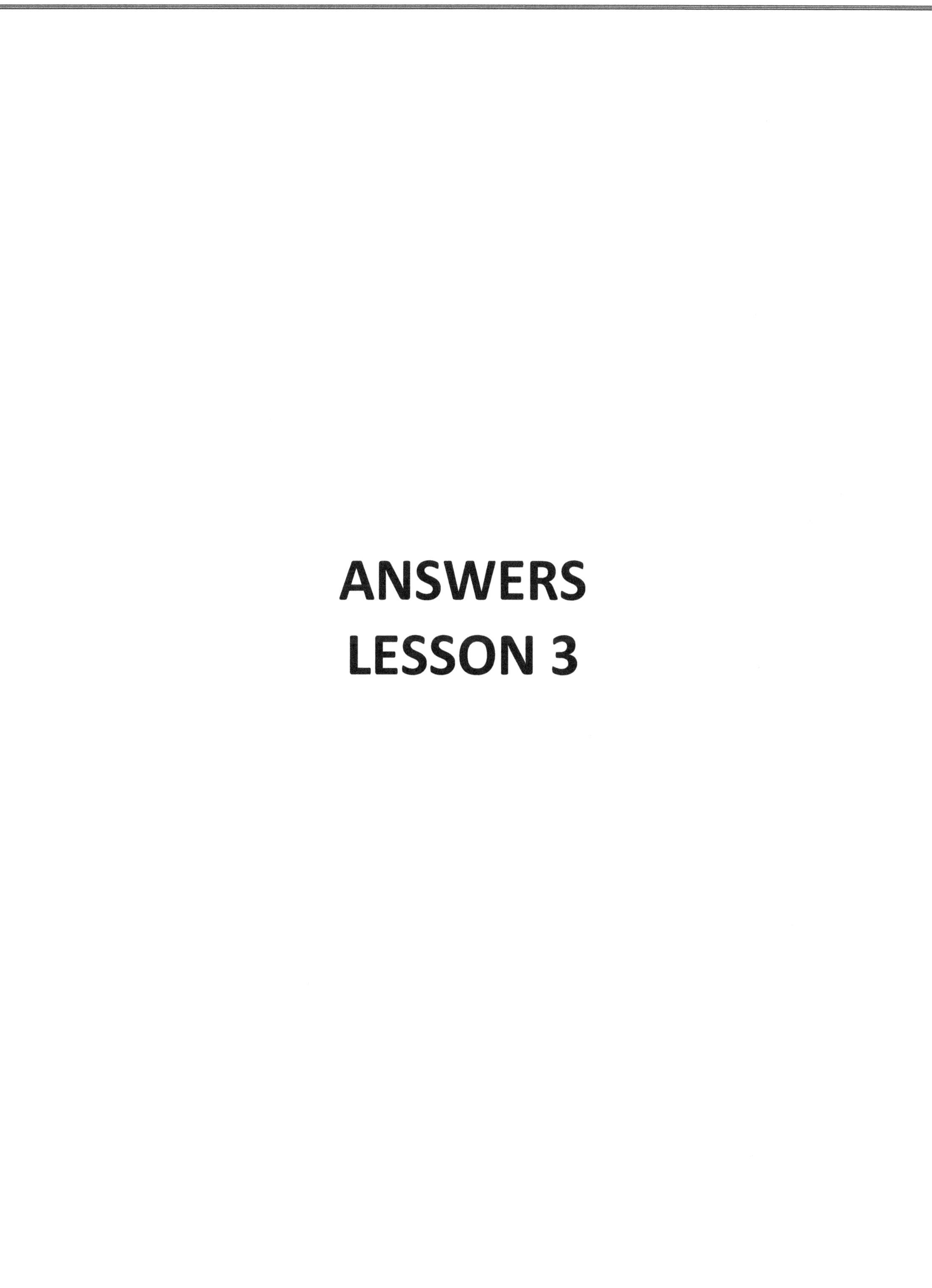

ANSWERS
LESSON 3

Answers to Lesson 3

Answers to Analyzing Data

1. 2018 Appx. $200
2. 2016 Appx. $14,000
3. 2019 Appx. $42,000

Net Profit/Loss
(-$13,200.00)
(-$8,400.00)
$700.00
$10,500.00

Answers to Logical Sequence

10,000	1,000	100	10	100	1,000	10,000	100,000	1,000,000	Remove 1 zero, then add 1 zero
750	725	700	675	650	625	600	575	550	Subtract 25 each time
20	22	26	32	40	50	62	76	92	Add, 2, then 4, then 6, then 8, 10, 12, 14, 16
15	30	60	120	240	480	960	1920	3840	Double the number each time

Answers to Logical Riddles

1. An Exterminator
2. He was born in room 1955
3. The Letter 'T'
4. He was the minister performing the ceremonies

Answers to Riddles-Overall Brain Challenge

1.) Eve promised to **turn over a new leaf**
2.) A **wise-quacker**
3.) Because it's **too far to walk**
4.) Put **clothes-pin on his nose**
5.) An **Electrician**
6.) On their **heads**
7.) By the number of **bugs** in his **teeth**
8.) A space **capsule**
9.) **TON**
10.) **Misery Loves Company**

Math Skills Review -3

52	68	10	61	27
11 r2	18	3 r5	94	4
251	352	216	476	436
371	320	393	305	240

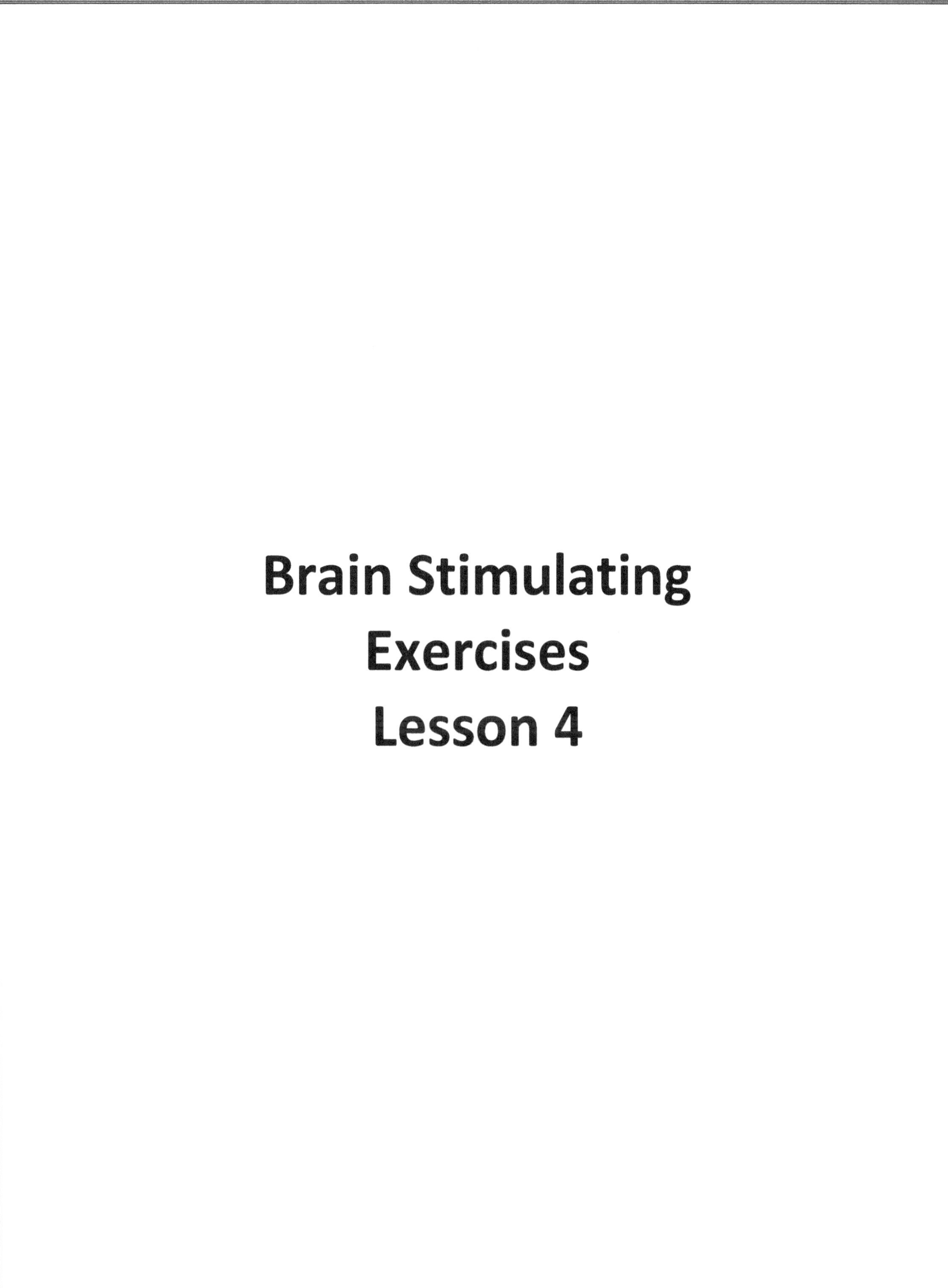

Brain Stimulating
Exercises
Lesson 4

<u>Reminder Page</u>

Don't forget to check off the following after you complete them today:

____ **Exercise**

____ **Prayer/Meditation**

____ **Self-Affirmations**

<u>SELF-AFFIRMATIONS</u>

What I do does not determine my worth.

I am worthy of love and respect.

I love myself and others.

I am loved by those who are important to me.

I am safe and protected by God.

I refuse to allow my mind to worry.

I am grateful for the life I have been given.

LESSON 4: Research & Discussion Sheet-The Brain that Writes

Whether you are a professional basketball player jumping and dunking or a writer working on your next great book, the brain activity that takes place during these activities is very similar.

Research in the area of neuroscience has been revealing some very interesting outcomes in the area of creative writing.

Neuroscientists use fMRI scanners to track the activity taking place in the brains of writers, and not just the professional authors, but all writers.

A team of researchers, led by Martin Lotze of the University of Greifswald in Germany, used scanners to "observe a broad network of regions in the brain working together as people wrote various stories." (Zimmer, 2014)

Some interesting finds have come out of this study.

First, experienced writers had intense brain activity in the same area of the brain that researchers would see in highly trained musicians and athletes. The greatest outcome of this study is that it gave the scientists a much better understanding of the important role creative writing plays in strengthening cognitive function.

Much of the writing we do in our BrainFlex workbooks is similar to the writing Dr. Lotze used in his study, including the activities that require 'brainstorming'.

Certain areas of the brain only become active when we 'brainstorm' and use the imagination to write. Even more beneficial to the brain is using visualization when we are writing. Seeing things with the 'mind's eye' stimulates an entirely different area of the brain.

When we engage in these types of activities, we are giving our brain an amazing workout, and the 'feel good' chemicals that are released when we accomplish something is just icing on the cake!

(healthy cake of course :)

References

Zimmer, C. (2014, June 20). *This is Your Brain on Writing* . Retrieved from New York Times:
https://www.nytimes.com/2014/06/19/science/researching-the-brain-of-writers.html

Exercise: Creativity ~ Imagination ~ Writing ~ Expression

Read the paragraph below, then exercise your creativity to develop
the story further. Explain the neighbor's plan in detail and don't forget
to engage your imagination.

Ben and Bella discovered that their neighbors have been plotting
and planning something over the past two years. Although they
aren't certain of the details, Ben believes they will act soon.

Fine Arts: Poetry ~ Expression/Creative Thinking/Vocabulary

Carefully and thoughtfully read the poem below. Cross out any misspelled words and write the correctly spelled word above it. Once you're finished, read the poem again, complete the related activity on the following page.

I look to the clouds and await once again,

To feel warmth on my face, to feel some piece deep within.

"Where is the ligt", I scream out the front door,

But not a rey can be found, not on the walls or the floor.

It is maddening, this grey, dimly lit, life that I live,

It seams the sky has not one spek of light left to give.

My thoughts start to wonder, as I fall back in my chair,

Losing myself, I gaze through the window and stair.

Thinking and pondering…when did my life start to change?

Do others search for the same, or am I going insain?

This discontantment…it seems to chase good things away,

Leaving a void in there place, now filled with feelings of grey.

As I sat in this daze, cuddeled down deep in my chair,

Eyes still fixed on the window; I sat twirling my hare.

Wandering what I was missing, does anyone else see the light?

I slowly drifted to sleep, as the day quickly became nite.

Fine Arts-Poetry ~ Expression/Creative Thinking

Creative thinking is an important part of what we do everyday.

One important outcome observed by researchers, is the connection between creative thinking and problem solving. Whenever we think about possibilities, especially that which is beyond 'the probable', we exercise the area of the brain that assists with problem solving. When we challenge the creative areas of our brain, whether we're using the imagination to understand a different perspective or to determine the thoughts and emotions behind various types of art, we are providing the brain with countless benefits.

1. After reading the poem on the previous page, what are your thoughts about its meaning? ______________________________

____

____

2. What do you feel may have been the mood of the writer?

What part of the poem makes you feel this way? ______________

____

____

3. The poem seems to leave us with a feeling that it's 'undone'. Exercise your creativity and bring the poem to a finish on the lines below, while attempting to maintain the pattern of the poem.

(Use your own thoughts and emotions, rather than those of the writer, and feel free to end the poem anyway you like!)

____

____

____

____

____

____

$2.50 + $7.00	$7.00 + $6.00	$8.50 + $5.00
$4.00 $5.50 + $6.00	$8.50 $2.50 + $7.00	$4.00 $5.50 + $6.00
$1.50 $9.50 + $7.50	$1.50 $3.00 + $9.00	$1.50 $9.50 + $7.50
579 332 272 + 519	169 654 861 + 389	169 490 231 + 572
4)17	9)58	9)44

Using Logic – Outside of the Box Problem Solving

1. Two mothers and two daughters, all went somewhere to eat.
   Each of them quite famished, from a day out in the heat.
   Then suddenly they realized that the food there wasn't free,
   So they decided on the pancakes, and said, "Please bring us three."
   So, tell me how each of them gobbled down one pancake whole,
   This rattling riddle on the brain will certainly take its toll.

   Explain how this could occur?
   ____

2. What is true? What is false?
   When I lay in this dimension
   I just turn and I toss
   Where am I? _______________________

3. You've heard me before, in a canyon, I think.
   When you called me, I answered before you could blink
   But who you were hearing? I ask with a wink
   What am I? _______________________

4. To your nose I will bring so much delight
   And Your eyes will enjoy me, especially at night.

   They measure my life, but only in hours,
   If left living too long, I am quickly devoured.
   What am I? _______________________

5. I wind up and throw...the ball soon out of sight,
   But it always comes back...at the speed of the light.
   It bounces off nothing...when I throw from the mound,
   There are no strings attached...and there's no one around.
   How does this happen? _______________________

6. I have many keys…they are all in a box
   They bring emotions to life…but they don't unlock locks.
   What am I? _______________________

Use this space for trivia, notes, math calculations
or to jot down a special memory.

92

ANSWERS
LESSON 4

Answers to-Fine Arts:Poetry ~ Expression/Creative Thinking

I look to the clouds and await once again,

To feel warmth on my face, to feel some **PEACE** deep within.

"Where is the **LIGHT**", I scream out the front door,

But not a **RAY** can be found, not on the walls or the floor.

It's maddening, this **GRAY**, dimly lit, life that I live,

It **SEEMS** the sky has not one **SPEC** of light left to give.

My thoughts start to **WANDER,** as I fall back in my chair,

Losing myself, I gaze through the window and **STARE.**

Thinking and pondering…when did my life start to change?

Do others search for the same, or am I going **INSANE?**

This **DISCONTENTMENT**…it seems to chase good things away,

Leaving a void in **THEIR** place, now filled with feelings of **GRAY**.

As I sat in this daze, now **CUDDLED** down deep in my chair,

Eyes still fixed on the window; I sat twirling my **HAIR.**

WONDERING, what I was missing, does anyone else see the light?

I slowly drifted to sleep, as the day quickly became **NIGHT.**

Answers to Lesson 4

Answers: Math Skills Review

$9.50	$13.00	$13.50
$15.50	$18.00	$15.50
$18.50	$13.50	$18.50
1702	2073	1462
4 r-1	6 r-4	4 r-8

_ Answers to Using Logic-Outside of the Box

1. The two mothers and two daughters were actually a grandmother, a mother and a daughter…but they could still be described as two mothers and two daughters, since the mother is both a mother and a daughter.

2. In a dream ---dreaming---dreamworld

3. I am YOUR ECHO

4. I am a CANDLE

5. Because he is throwing the ball straight up in the air, and gravity is bringing it right back to him.

6. I am a PIANO

Use this space to doodle, make a few notes,
or to write about a special memory.

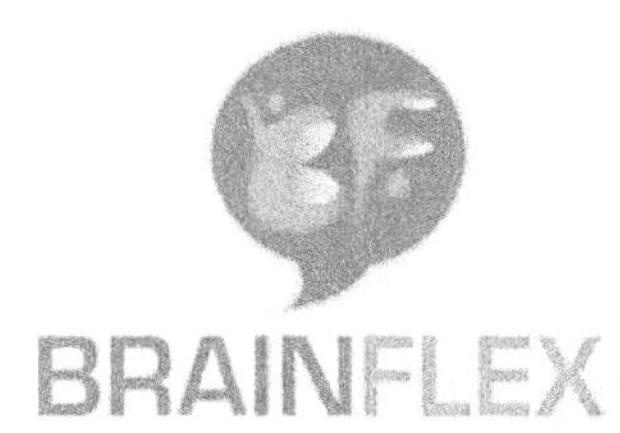

WEEK THREE

NUTRITIONAL RECIPE

Contributing to a healthier brain & body

The health benefits in the recipe's ingredients will vary with each individual and depend heavily upon each person's level of commitment to making healthy life-style choices on a consistent basis.

Avocado Egg Toast

INGREDIENTS

¼ AVOCADO

1 TSP. FRESH SALSA

1 BOILED EGG (SLICED)

1 DASH OF SALT

1 DASH OF PEPPER

1 SLICE OF SPROUTED WHOLE GRAIN BREAD (TOASTED)
(Another good choice is fresh sour dough bread or gluten free bread.)

HEALTH BENEFITS OF AVOCADOS

Avocados are full of brain healthy fats mono-unsaturated fatty acids, which are necessary for the heart as well.

Avocados have been shown to help lower cholesterol.

Avocados are high in fiber, which contributes to digestive health. (Digestive health plays a major role in brain health.)

The healthy fats in avocados help your body absorb nutrients from other healthy plant-based foods you may consume.

Health Benefits of Organic Whole Grain Bread

-High in fiber, which contributes to better digestive health.

-Contains Vitamin B, Niacin, Thiamine and Folate

-Contains Minerals, such as Zinc, Iron, & Magnesium

-Contains several compounds that act as antioxidants

   *These include phytic acid, lignin & sulfur

-Whole grains deliver many types of plant compounds that help the body battle disease.

   *These include lignans, stanols and sterols.

Health Benefits in 1 Egg:
- Vitamin A: 6% of the RDA
- Folate: 5% of the RDA
- Vitamin B5: 7% of the RDA
- Vitamin B12: 9% of the RDA
- Vitamin B2: 15% of the RDA
- Phosphorus: 9% of the RDA
- Selenium: 22% of the RDA
- Eggs also contain vitamin D, vitamin E, vitamin K, vitamin B6, calcium & zinc

Learn more about a few of these vitamins & minerals on the following slides.

Selenium: Eggs contain 22% (RDA)

-One purpose of this mineral is to make sure certain body processes work correctly.

-Selenium is used to battle diseases related to blood vessels, cholesterol, diabetes, asthma, eczema, and some cancers.

These cancers include prostate, colon, rectum, stomach, esophagus, lung, ovary, bladder & skin.

This is only a partial list of the benefits.

<u>**Vitamin B2: Eggs contain 15% *(RDA)***</u>

<u>Vitamin B2 is Riboflavin.</u>

-This vitamin is used to battle migraine headaches, muscle cramps, carpal tunnel syndrome, and various eye conditions, such as cataracts and glaucoma.

-Riboflavin also gives the immune system a boost and helps the body maintain healthy hair, skin & nails.

-Some research studies have shown that vitamin B2 can help slow the aging process and battle Alzheimer's disease as well as other diseases that cause dementia.

<u>**Vitamin B-12: Eggs contain 9% *(RDA)***</u>

This is a water-soluble vitamin that is important to nerve function, the formation of red blood cells, and the production of DNA.

B-12 helps the body battle heart and blood vessel disease and has been associated with dementia prevention.

> *This is because a deficiency in B-12 has been shown to effect cognitive function.*

Use this space to doodle, make notes,
or to jot down a special memory.

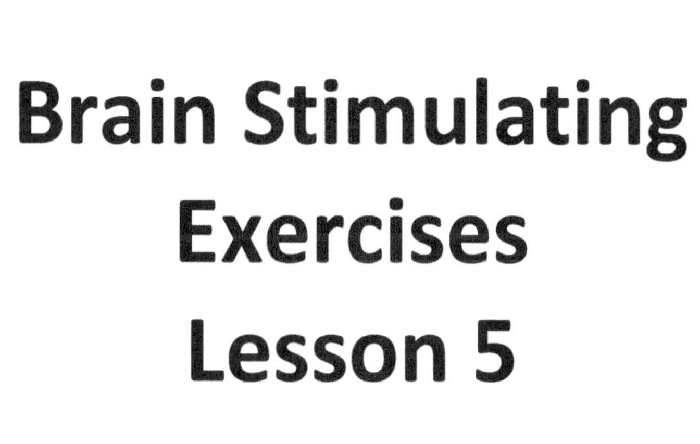

Brain Stimulating
Exercises
Lesson 5

<u>Reminder Page</u>

Don't forget to check off the following after you complete them today:

____ **Exercise**

____ **Prayer/Meditation**

____ **Self-Affirmations**

<u>SELF-AFFIRMATIONS</u>

I believe in personal growth, so I love to learn.

I am brave and courageous.

I am curious and creative.

God has given me a beautiful, sound mind.

I have a youthful spirit and mind.

Sharing my life experiences is one way I will contribute to the world.

Most of us think playing brain games is just another way to have fun. Of course, that's true, but it's so much more. It's having fun with brain benefits! Answering questions, solving problems, thinking outside of the box, etc., all provide wonderful benefits for the brain…and the beautiful thing is, you don't even have to be the one that answers the question to receive the benefits.

Why? Because you are still thinking, learning, writing and communicating, which are all great ways to work out your "mind's muscle". However, when you do answer a question, whether it's through recall or solving a problem, you are strengthening your neural pathways.

How? Well, I'm sure you've heard the phrase, "Use it or lose it." This applies to more than just the muscles in our body, it holds true for our brain as well. Challenging brain activities, such as those included in 'The BrainFlex Workbook', are to our brains, as lifting weights is to our muscles. When we lift weights, it pushes our muscles past their limits, but the result is a stronger body. When we work hard to solve problems, recall answers to trivia, think to create, etc., we are pushing our brain to do more than normal.

A Note about TV. Engaging in activities that stimulate the brain requires so MUCH more brain power than watching television, which, by the way, can actually cause atrophy in the brain. If you must watch TV, limit your time, especially if you're watching the news. (It's best to watch something educational.) In addition, it's important to guard your mind when choosing what to watch on television and not allow your eyes and ears to take in too much of the 'negative'. It takes work and discipline to stay positive and if we guard our minds, we are already half way there. Research continually shows that positive thinking is a key component to a healthy brain, but it's something that requires discipline and intentionality.

Last, it's natural for most people to lean towards the negative. For example, you don't have to teach a child to say no, to lie, or to get angry when they don't get their way, it's innate in our humanness. Staying positive and replacing negative thoughts with positive ones takes commitment. However, just like any discipline, it gets easier with time and it's worth the fight. Remember, a little progress each day adds up…and becomes the difference maker.

Word-Language Exercise

Determine the answers to these tricky word challenges,
then write them on the line provided in each box.

Once **5:00 pm** _____ _____ ___ _____	**Mad** **Mad U Mad** **Mad** _____ _____ _____	**Long** **Do** _____ _____
TheALLfamily _____ _____ _____ _____	**Head ac he** A _ _ _ _ _ _ _ _ _ _ _ _ _ _	**Hahandnd** _____ _____
Lang4uage _____ _____	Give Get Give Get _____ Give Get _____ Give Get _____	**Go it it it it** _____ _____ _____
Na **T** _ _ _ **Na** **F** _ _ _ **Fish**	k c u _____ t s _____	**YYYYYYYYYY** **Guy** _____ _____
Rest **You're** _____ ' _ _____ _____	Head **LO** Heels **VE** _____ _____ _____ _____	**M Just You E** _____ _____ _____ _____

<u>CREATIVE DRAWING</u>

For years, many of the typical 'IQ' tests were not able to measure creativity, which is a vital part of the thinking process. Fortunately, this was recognized and exercises similar to what you see below were added to these tests.

In each of the boxes below, start with the image given and create your own picture. This activity is a great way to engage your creative side, while also exercising your imagination, (and both are important components to problem solving).

Do your best to 'make a statement' with each drawing.

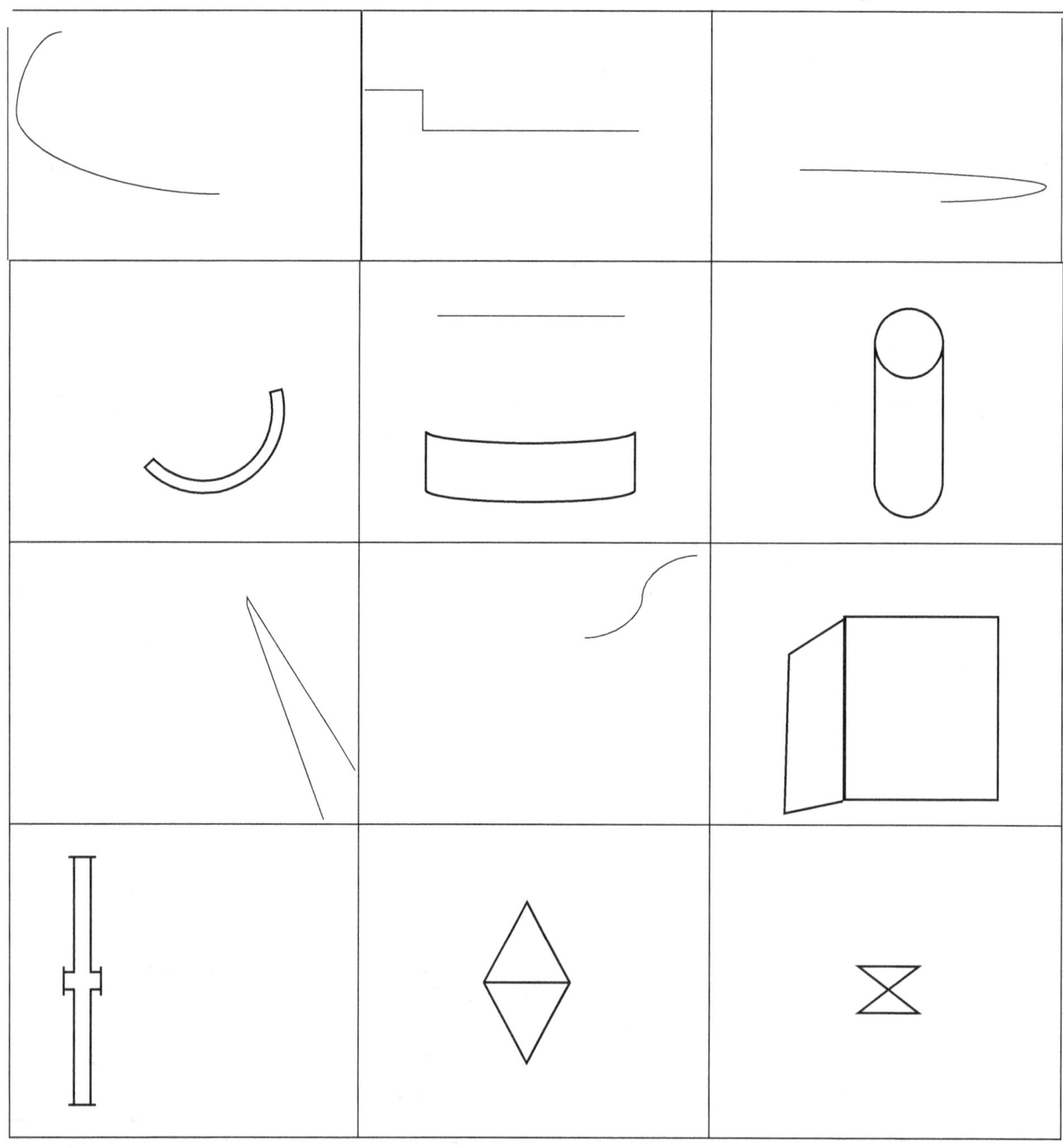

<u>Thought Process ~ Speed</u>

Read each question below and write down the first answer that comes to your mind, then move on to the next question as quickly as possible.
(This exercise is designed to challenge your processing speed.)

1) What famous person would you like to interview?

   ____

2) Name something you could eat 10 of in one minute._______________

3) What is something that most people try to avoid? _________________

4) Name something you would love to do in a crowd of people.

   ____

5) Name something accountants may dislike about their job.

   ____

6) What is something a non-productive adult does often?

   ____

7) Name something you could buy with .75 cents.

   ____

8) Name something on which you should walk carefully.

   ____

9) Name something associated with Frank Sinatra.

   ____

10) Name something made with flour.

   ____

11) Name something stored in a shed.

   ____

12) Name a U.S. state that has a lot of mountains.

   ____

Math Word Problems

1. After experiencing severe knee pain for several weeks, Fred finally went to the doctor. During his examination, his doctor expressed concern over Fred's weight, warning him that surgery was inevitable if he didn't lose weight.

On February 1, Frank weighed 227 pounds. His doctor told him that he wanted him to get his weight down to 195 lbs., 10 months from that day.
By July 1st, Fred had lost 20 pounds, so he decided to go on a cruise July 7th through the 11th, to celebrate. Unfortunately, he gained 7 pounds on his cruise, and by the end of the month, he had gained an additional 13lbs.!
In what month will Fred be expected to weigh 195 lbs.? _______________

On February 1st, the doctor told Fred he had to lose _______lbs. in 10 months.

How much did Fred weigh on July 11th? _________________

By the end of July, Fred gained an additional 20 lbs., He now only has ________ months to lose _____________ lbs.

What is the average number of pounds Fred will have to lose each month in order to stay within the time frame set by the doctor? _________/month.

____

2. Jerry is getting ready to take his grandsons on a camping trip and they are planning to leave at 5:00 the next morning. If the campsite is 360 miles away and Jerry drives 60 mph, how many hours will they be on the road? ____________

If they plan to leave at 5:00 am, what time would Jerry and his grandsons arrive to the campsite? _______________

Jerry's grandsons want to stop for breakfast, which will add 1 hour and 45 minutes to their trip. Now what time will they arrive to the campsite? _________

____

3. Clara is getting ready to go shopping for her grandchildren. She will be purchasing each of them a birthday gift, as she likes to buy all the birthday gifts for the year in one shopping trip. Clara and her husband George had three children together and they both had three children before they married. Six of the children are married and each couple has two children of their own, but the rest of their children are still single.

    How many children do Clara and George have all together? _______________
    How many gifts will Clara need to purchase for her grandchildren? ________
    How many people are in George and Clara's family all together? _________

ANSWERS
LESSON 5

<u>Answers to 'Concentration with Language and Memory</u>

Once upon a time	Mad for you (mad four U)	Long overdue
All in the Family	Splitting headache	Hand in hand
Foreign Language (four in language)	Forgive and forget (four give – four get)	Go for it (go four it)
Tuna Fish (two 'na' fish)	Stuck up	Wise guy (y's guy)
You're under arrest (you're under a rest)	Head over heels in love	Just you and me (just you in me)

1. In what month will Fred be expected to weigh 195 lbs.? **NOVEMBER**
On February 1st, the doctor told Fred he had to lose **32 lbs**. in 10 months.
How much did Fred weigh on July 11th? **207 lbs**
By the end of July, Fred had gained 20 lbs., He now only has **4** months to lose **32 lbs.**
What is the average number of pounds Fred will have to lose each month in order to stay within the time frame set by the doctor? **8lbs**/month.

2. Jerry is getting ready to take his grandsons on a camping trip and they are planning to leave at 5:00 the next morning. If the campsite is 360 miles away and Jerry drives 60 mph, how many hours will they be on the road? **6 hrs.**
If they plan to leave at 5:00 am, what time would Jerry and his grandsons arrive to the campsite? **11 am**
Jerry's grandsons want to stop for breakfast, which will add 1 hour and 45 minutes to their trip. Now what time will they arrive to the campsite? **12:45 pm**

3. How many children do Clara and George have all together? **9** (3+3+3)
How many gifts will Clara need to purchase for her grandchildren? **12 gifts** (6 of their children each have 2 children, (6x2=12)
How many people are in George & Clara's family all together? **29**
(George & Clara-2) (their children-9) (6 of the 9 children are married, so add their spouses-6) (then add their grandchildren-12)---(2+9+6+12=29)

Answers to all other activities in the lesson will vary.

Brain Stimulating
Exercises
Lesson 6

<u>Reminder Page</u>

Don't forget to check off the following after you complete them today:

_____ **Exercise**

_____ **Prayer/Meditation**

_____ **Self-Affirmations**

Self-Affirmations

I am cherished and valuable.

No one in the world has my unique DNA.

I deserve to be happy, so I choose to be happy.

I'm okay with vulnerability and I want to be real.

I talk about the lessons life has taught me with the next generation.

Today is going to be a beautiful day.

LESSON 6: The Power of a Positive Attitude

Positive people have a mental and emotional attitude that is focused on the 'bright side'. They seem to go through life expecting good things to happen. You may think to yourself, 'Well, that's just how they are.'   It is true that some people tend to lean toward the 'silver lining', while others have the feeling that most good things are either too good to be true or they won't last. Regardless of which way your mental mindset may lean, it can change…if you want it to.

Most researchers agree that negative and positive mindsets are learned behaviors, which means they can be unlearned. So, when you (or someone you know) says, "It's just the way I am," keep in mind that it's a choice. With that being said…change is hard, and the older we get, the more difficult change can be. The cliché', 'you can't teach an old dog new tricks', does not have to be true for you, but that doesn't mean it won't take some effort.

Before we discuss this any further, let me address the skeptics. There are those who are convinced that positive thinking is nonsense and may even be tempted to thumb their noses up at the thought of becoming a more positive person. However, there is now an overwhelming amount of scientific evidence that confirms the positive effects that a good attitude and hopeful thinking can have on the brain and body. This is even more effective when we take it a step further and become intentional about using positive words and keeping anger and bitterness out of our lives.

We often discuss the benefits our brain and body receive from a life committed to positive thinking, so let's talk about another benefit. For example, positive people have a unique body language that can subconsciously make others feel more positive. Of course, the kind words, that are typically a part of the positive person's vocabulary can also make those around them feel good.

What's usually the natural outcome for such a person? They are never short of friends. People are drawn to them, which only feeds the positive person's positivity! It typically takes about 63 days of intentional and purposeful commitment to replace negative thoughts and words with positive ones. (Try to do this the moment these thoughts come to your mind or before they come out of your mouth.) You'll be surprised at the difference this makes in your day, and in your relationships.

BrainFlex® Wellness©

Reading Comprehension and Recall Exercise

After reading the story, answer the questions below, doing your best to challenge your recall by avoiding looking back at the story.

Mary Schneider is 32 years old. She married Dave 10 years ago in Jefferson City, Missouri. Dave is an engineer at McDonnell Douglas in St. Louis, where they now reside. Mary works in downtown St. Louis as a CPA for a large accounting firm. Every Friday night is 'Girls' night out', and also one of Mary's favorite nights of the week. Dave and Mary stay very active and have a regular travel schedule. The first Saturday of every month, they visit Mary's nephew, Jake, who lives in Bixby, Oklahoma. Jake is 23 and recently graduated from Evangel University. The last Saturday of every month, they visit Mary's sisters, Gail and Gloria, who live in Chicago. Every Wednesday, Mary & Dave attend Bible Study at a local church, where they enjoy learning more about God.

1. Dave's last name is most likely to be...______________________________

2. How old was Mary when she married Dave? ________________

3. How many siblings does Mary have? ________

4. On Saturday, May 2nd, Dave & Mary will be traveling to visit her ____________ who lives in ________________ ______________.

5. On Wednesday, May 9th, Dave & Mary will be heading to a ______________ ________________ at their local ________________.

6. On Saturday, May 27th, Dave and Mary plan on traveling to ____________________ to visit her ____________________.

7. What occurs every Friday night? _______________________________

8. What are the names of Mary's sisters? ______________ and

____

9. Where did Jake go to college?______________ ______________

10. Mary's brother called her to ask if she could help him file his ________ return, which she was able to do with ease because she is a

________.

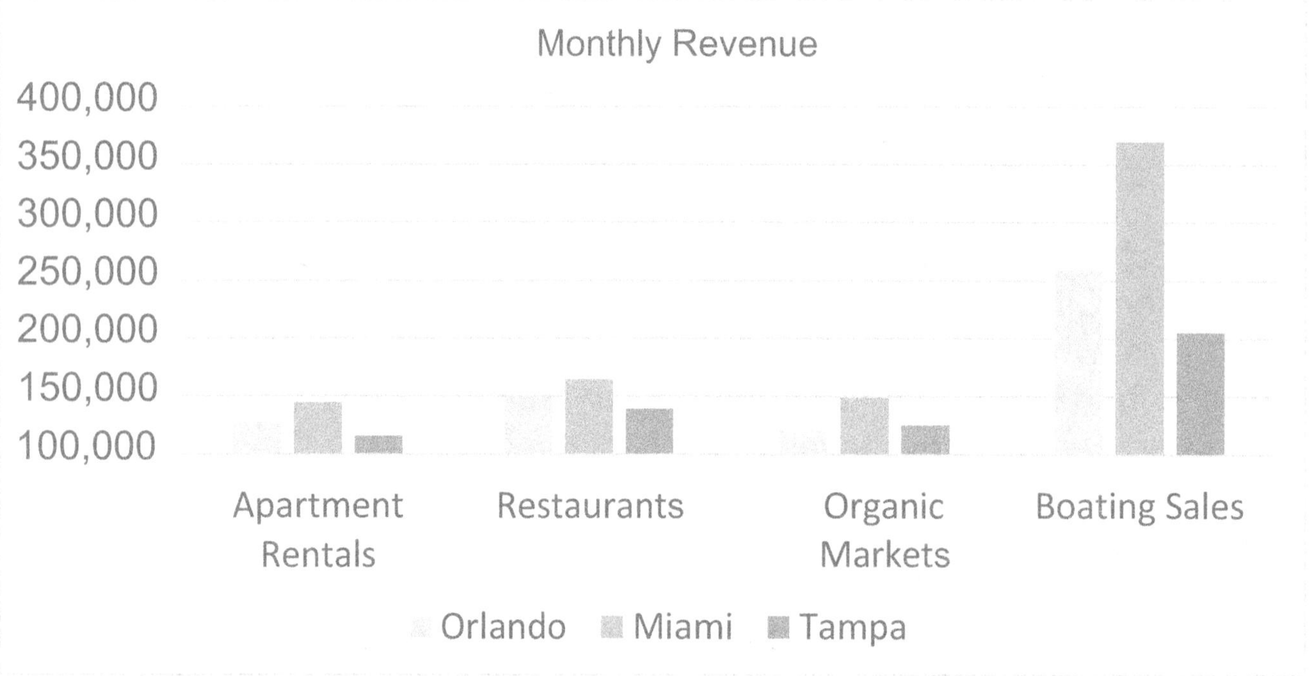

Monthly Operational Costs	Orlando	Miami	Tampa
R & K Apartment Rentals	$ 26,000	$ 35,000	$ 22,000
R & K Restaurants	$ 65,000	$ 70,000	$ 60,000
R & K Organic Markets	$ 36,000	$ 53,000	$ 41,000
R & K Boating Sales	$ 71,000	$ 104,000	$ 56,000

A. Ken & Ramone are selling the **restaurants** they own in each of the Florida cities above, but want to do an overview of the monthly net profit earned by each restaurant for the purchaser(s). Review the monthly **revenue** recorded on the chart at the very top of the page, (*these will be 'approximate' numbers*), then **subtract the monthly operational costs** (shown in the graph directly below the chart) to determine the **net profit** earned by each restaurant.

Orlando: Net Profit: $ ______________
Miami: Net Profit: $ ______________
Tampa: Net Profit: $ ______________

B. Ken and Ramone are considering selling all their companies located in Miami. However, they want to be sure the performance of the companies in Orlando and Tampa are solid. From the chart at the very top of the page, determine the **total** '*approximate*' monthly revenue generated by the six remaining companies, (*excluding the restaurants*). $___________

C. Determine the net profit earned by:
Miami Apartment Rentals $________

Charts, Graphs, Logic and Reason
Use the chart/graph to answer the questions in each box.

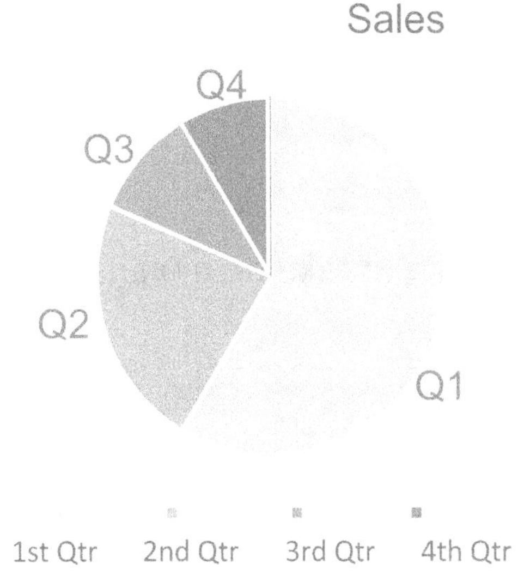

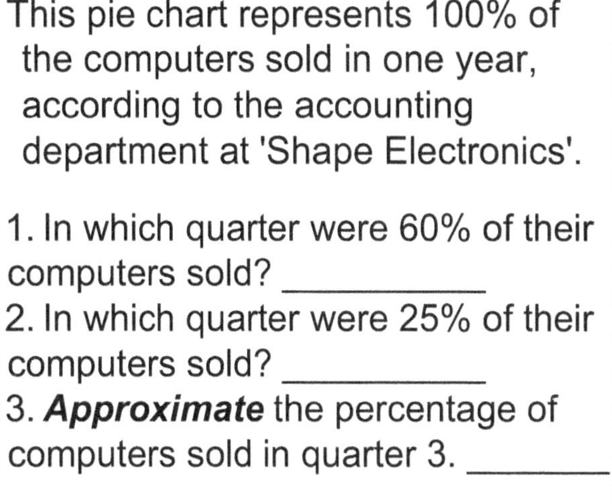

This pie chart represents 100% of the computers sold in one year, according to the accounting department at 'Shape Electronics'.

1. In which quarter were 60% of their computers sold? ___________
2. In which quarter were 25% of their computers sold? ___________
3. **Approximate** the percentage of computers sold in quarter 3. _________

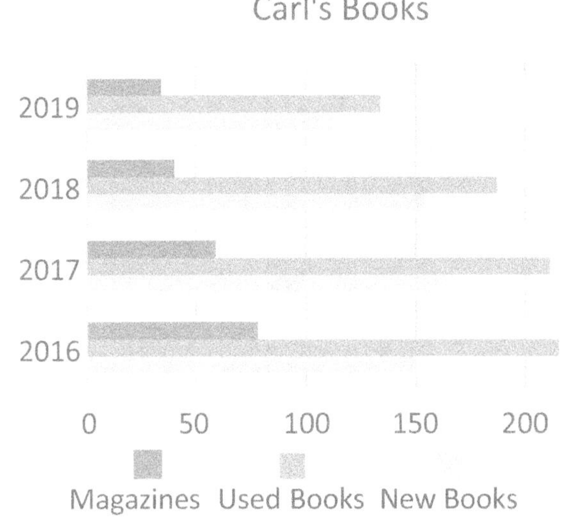

The bar chart represents the sales for 'Carl's Books' over a 4-year period.
1. In ______ (yr.) Carl's sales for used books were the highest. Approximately how many did he sell? _________
2. In ______ (yr.) Carl sold the lowest number of magazines, selling only_____
3. In _______ (yr.) Carl had the highest new book sales overall, selling approximately ________ new books.
4. What trend do you see with Carl's business? ______________________________

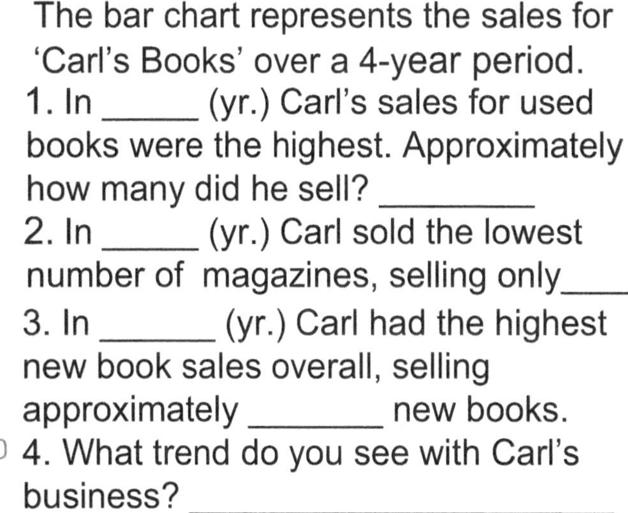

The line chart represents the sales for Rye's Ford Dealer during quarter 1.
1. The unusual car sales spike during the month of ____________ resulted in the sale of _____ cars.
2. ____________ had the lowest sales during the month of _____________ selling only ______ *(number)*
3. In the space below, next to each month, write the vehicles with the highest sales and the amount sold.
January: ______________ - ______
February: ______________ - ______
March: ______________ - ______

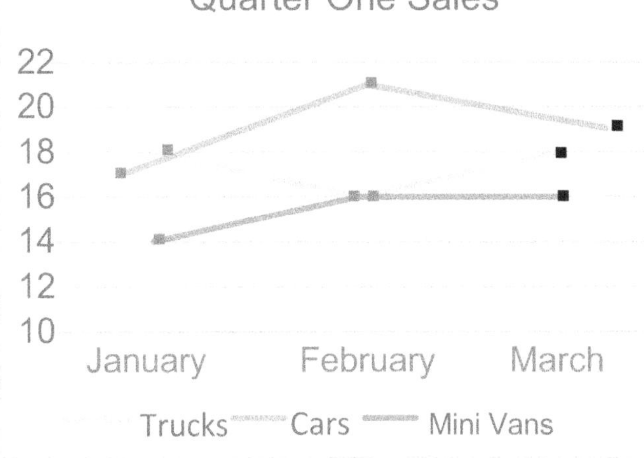

Thought Processing Speed: Answer the following with the first thoughts that come to your mind. (Imagine you're working against the clock!)

1) Name 3 things you shouldn't advertise in the paper.

    1_______________________________________

    2_______________________________________

    3_______________________________________

2) Name 3 musical instruments that are too big to take on a plane.

    1_______________________________________

    2_______________________________________

    3_______________________________________

3) Name 3 things people typically save.

    1_______________________________________

    2_______________________________________

    3_______________________________________

4) Name 3 things you always do before going to bed.

    1_______________________________________

    2_______________________________________

    3_______________________________________

5) Name 3 things people do to get on the boss' good side.

    1_______________________________________

    2_______________________________________

    3_______________________________________

6) Name 3 things men usually carry in their pockets.

    1_______________________________________

    2_______________________________________

    3_______________________________________

ANSWERS
LESSON 6

Answers: Reading Comprehension and Recall

1. Dave's last name is most likely to be... *Schneider*
2. How old was Mary when she married Dave? *22*
3. How many sisters does Mary have? *2*
4. On Saturday, May 2nd, Dave & Mary will be traveling to visit her *brother, Jake* who lives in *Bixby, Oklahoma*
5. On Wednesday, May 9th, Dave & Mary will be heading to a *Bible Study* at their local *church*
6. On Saturday, May 27th, Dave and Mary plan on traveling to *Chicago* to visit her *sisters*.
7. What occurs every Friday night? *girls night out*
8. What are the names of Mary's sisters? *Gail, Gloria*
9. Where did Jake go to college? *Evangel University*
10. Mary's brother called her to ask if she could help him file his *tax* return, which she was able to do with ease, since she is a *CPA*

Answers: Ken & Ramone's Empire Management

A. Ken & Ramone are selling the **restaurants** they own in each of the Florida cities above, but want to do an overview of the monthly net profit earned by each restaurant for the purchaser. Review the monthly revenue recorded on the chart at the top of the page, (*these will be 'approximate' numbers*), then subtract the monthly operational costs shown in the graph directly below the chart, to determine the net profit earned by the **R & K Restaurants** in all three cities.

**Revenue – Operating Costs = Net Profit*

Orlando: Net Profit: $ *85,000* $150 K - $65K = $85K
Miami: Net Profit: $ *90,000* $160K - $70K= $90K
Tampa: Net Profit: $ *80,000* $140K - $60K = $80K

B. Ken and Ramone are considering selling all their companies located in Miami. However, they want to be sure the performance of the companies in Orlando and Tampa are solid. From the chart at the top of the page, determine the total 'approximate' monthly revenue generated by the six remaining companies **$945,000**

C. $130 K - $35 K= **$95 K**

A. (Math)
Orlando Restaurant Revenue ($150,000) – Operating Costs ($65,000) = $85,000
Miami Restaurant Revenue ($160,000) – Operating Costs ($70,000) = $90,000
Tampa Restaurant Revenue ($140,000) – Operating Costs (60,000) = $80,000
B. (Math) Total approximate revenue from all Orlando and Tampa restaurants
(excluding the restaurants)
Total revenue for Apartments, Organic Market, Boating Sales in...
Orlando: $125K + $120K + $255K = $500
Tampa: $115K + $125K + $205K = $445

Where questions include the word 'approximate', answers may vary slightly.

Answers: Charts, Graphs, Logic and Reason

This pie chart represents 100% of the computers sold in one year, according to the accounting departments at 'Shape Electronics'.

1. In which quarter were 60% of their computers sold? **Q-1**
2. In which quarter were 25% of their computers sold? **Q-2**
3. Approximate the percentage of computers sold in quarter 3. **8%** appx.

The bar chart represents the sales for 'Carl's Books' over a 4-year period.
1. In **2016** (yr.) Carl's sales for used books were the highest. Approximately how many did he sell? **215**
2. In **2019** (yr.) Carl sold the lowest number of magazines, selling only **40**
3. In **2017** (yr.) Carl had the highest new book sales overall, selling approximately **170** new books.
4. What trend do you see with Carl's business? **reduced sales each year.**

The line chart represents the sales for Rye's Ford Dealer during quarter 1.
1. The unusual car sales spike during the month of **Feb.** resulted in the sale of **21** cars.
2. **Mini-Van** had the lowest sales during the month of **Jan.** selling only **14** (number)
3. In the space below, next to each month, write the vehicles with the highest sales and the amount sold.
January: **Trucks** - **18**
February: **Cars** - **21**
March: **Cars** - **19**

Use this space to make notes, or to jot down
an important lesson life has taught you.

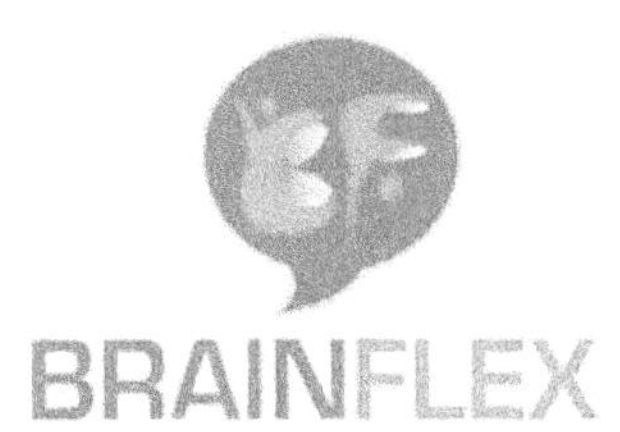

WEEK FOUR

NUTRITIONAL RECIPE

Contributing to a healthier brain & body

The health benefits in the recipe's ingredients will vary with each individual and depend heavily upon each person's level of commitment to making healthy life-style choices on a consistent basis.

White Bean Caprese Salad

Serves: 6

- 1 - 15oz. can of *Great Northern Organic Bean's* , drained and rinsed
- 2 cups quartered cherry tomatoes
- 2 ½ oz. fresh mozzarella, cut into 1" cubes
- 1 garlic clove, finely minced
- ¼ tsp. salt
- pepper to taste
- 10 fresh basil leaves, chopped,
- 2 tsp. olive oil
- 2 tsp. balsamic glaze

Instructions	Combine beans and tomatoes in large bowl.
	Add basil and mozzarella - stir.
	Mix in garlic, salt, and pepper.
	Drizzle with olive oil and balsamic glaze.

Health Benefits: **Northern Beans**	• Packed with protein, which promotes healthy muscles, skin and other organs, while also helping the body heal and maintain fluid.
	• Protein keeps you full and satisfied, reducing the urge to snack on unhealthy foods from the pantry.
	• Very high in fiber, providing your digestive system with much of the recommended daily allowance.

Health Benefits:

Tomatoes

- Contain natural anti-inflammatory properties (Inflammation can cause joint pain, digestive issues and brain fog, just to name a few.)

- Lycopene in tomatoes has been shown to be beneficial to bone health, especially in women.

- Nutrient Dense: Contains vitamin C, vitamin K, Calcium, and some beta-carotene as well.

- Packed full of anti-oxidants, which help the body fight off illnesses and disease.

Health Benefits:

Garlic

- Contains antimicrobial, antiviral, and antibacterial properties, which fight infection and reduce the risk of food borne illnesses.

- Plays a vital role in the battle against inflammation in the body
- Can help the body naturally produce more white blood cells

- Has been shown to help battle **fatigue**

<table>
<tr><td>Health
Benefits:

Olive Oil</td><td>-Contains well-researched anti-inflammatory compounds

-Full of antioxidants, helping the body battle cell damaging free radicals

-Research studies have shown extra virgin olive oil can assist with the battle against depression, dementia and obesity.

-Olive oil is high in healthy fatty acids, which contribute to heart health and brain function.</td></tr>
</table>

Health Benefits: Mozzarella

B-12 - Mozzarella contains 38% of the RDA.
Research studies now reveal B-12 is beneficial to brain function.

-**Riboflavin** – (B-2)- Contains 17% of the RDA – Important to cell growth and assists with many of the body's natural processes.
-**Calcium** - Contains 51% of the RDA - Calcium is extremely important to bone health, especially for seniors, since bone density tends to decrease as we age.
-**Phosphorus** - Contains 35% of the RDA - This mineral assists the body with the absorption of Calcium.
-**Selenium** - 24% of the RDA – A powerful antioxidant which has been shown to support cognitive function and to boost immunity as well.

Use this space to make notes, or to jot down
an important lesson life has taught you.

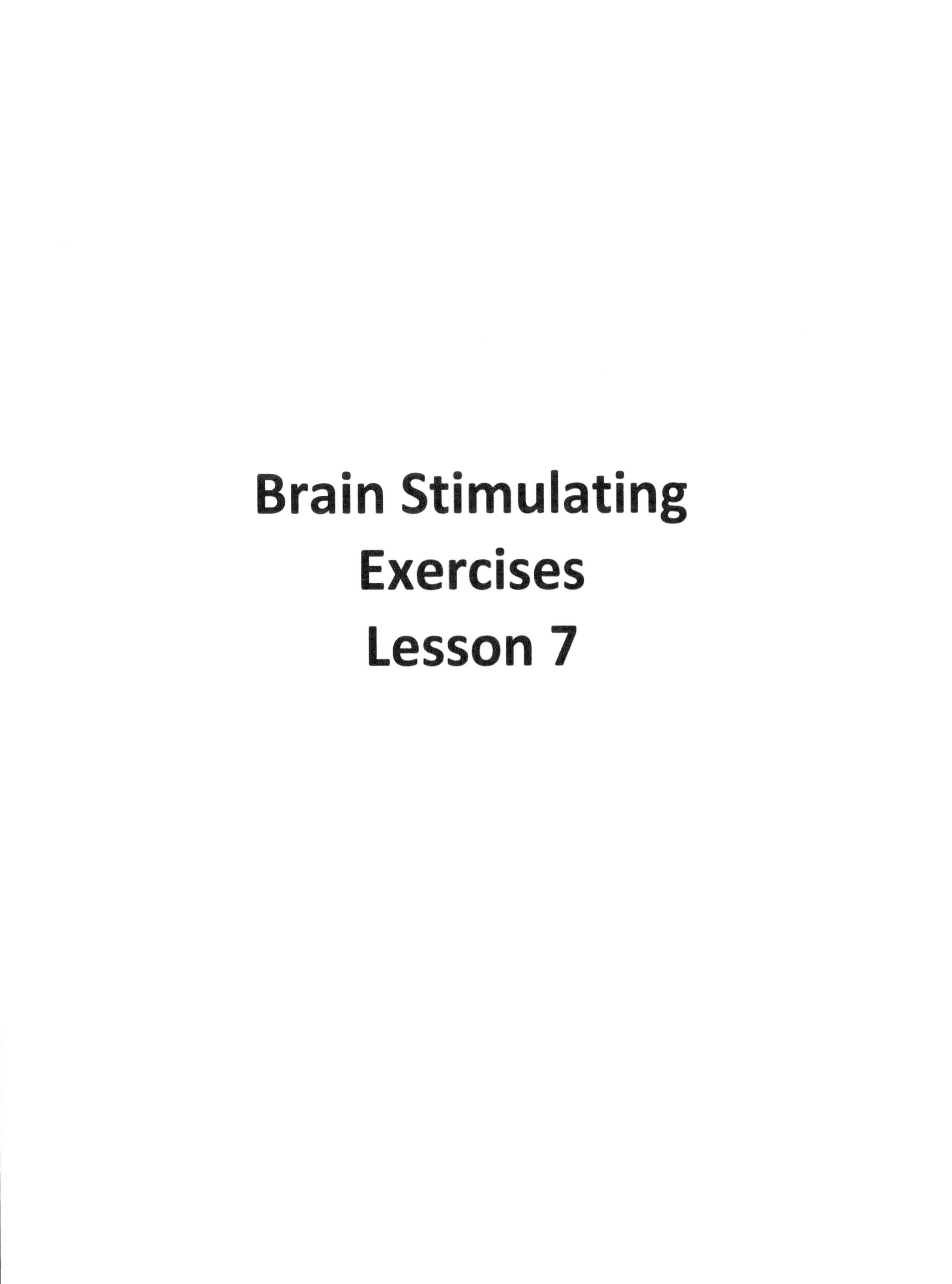

Brain Stimulating Exercises
Lesson 7

<u>Reminder Page</u>

Don't forget to check off the following after you complete them today:

_____ Exercise

_____ Prayer/Meditation

_____ Self-Affirmations

<u>SELF-AFFIRMATIONS</u>

I TAKE ACTION TO MAINTAIN MY INDEPENDENCE.

I AM FILLED WITH LOVE.

TODAY I CHOOSE TO RELEASE ALL ANGER.

MY MIND IS FREE OF NEGATIVITY.

I WILL ASSUME THE BEST WHEN I CONSIDER THE MOTIVES OF OTHERS.

LESSON 7: Mental Cross Training-Discussion Sheet

Have you heard of the term, cross fitness?

- Maybe you immediately think of the guy with the big muscles, but it simply means that you are attempting to make every area of the body fit by working out a variety of muscles.

- In the case of 'mental cross training', it means you are attempting to make every area of your brain fit by doing a variety of brain stimulating activities.

- When people are participating in cross training, they are engaging in various versions of physical fitness, each providing benefits to different parts of the body. (This may also include different sports.)
  - The outcome is an overall strengthening for the body, rather than just one or two areas.

- The activities in this workbook are designed in a similar way! You will continually experience a wide variety of challenges, such as trivia, problem solving, critical thinking, logic, reasoning and the 'stirring up' of the creative side with the use of imagination. In addition, you will have the opportunity to challenge your language and vocabulary skills and think outside of the box, (and draw outside of the lines). Many of these are tasks in which our brain typically doesn't engage…which is what makes it so beneficial.

- The life-long learning component included in the BrainFlex workbook exposes us to new and interesting information. These are just a few of the different types of exercises that work together to provide an amazing 'Cross-Training' workout for the brain.

References

Bourestan, K. (2017 , Novemember 7). *Benefits of Trivia Questions*. Retrieved from Mantelligence:
    https://www.mantelligence.com/benefits-of-trivia-questions/

Language and Vocab Centers – Attention to Detailed Instruction

Create as many words as possible using the letters below.

<u>Guidelines</u>: When using the letters in the graph to create a word, keep in mind that the letters must be touching, but they can go in any direction. Also, words must contain at least 3 letters. Each letter can only be used once in a word, but may be used again in another word.

H	A	B	I	V
R	I	E	O	O
E	I	M	O	N
O	E	A	T	R
D	E	G	U	T

___________________   ___________________   ___________________

___________________   ___________________   ___________________

___________________   ___________________   ___________________

___________________   ___________________   ___________________

___________________   ___________________   ___________________

___________________   ___________________   ___________________

___________________   ___________________   ___________________

___________________   ___________________   ___________________

<u>Creative Thinking for Problem Solving</u>

Think outside of the box to solve the following problems, then write the approapriate response in the space provided.

1. Ron stumbled upon a treasure chest that had been washed up on the shore. He could see that it was full of treasure, but it was also full of sand. Suddenly a genie appeared and told Ron that he could have the entire chest if he could figure out a way to carry it home by himself. The chest was so heavy that Ron couldn't lift it more than an inch off the ground. He reached for his cell phone, and realized he had left it at home...three miles away. The genie went on to say, "You may not take anything out of the chest; however, you can put whatever you want in it. **What Advice would you give to Ron?**___________________

____

2. Andrea walked into the house and flipped on the lights, but nothing happened. She knew there had been a storm but had no idea that the electricity had gone out in the entire city. She reached into the kitchen drawer and pulled out a box of matches, but there was only one left. She isn't sure what she should light first, a candle, her fireplace, or something else. **What should Andrea light first?**

____

3. Virgil quickly walked by the kitchen, then suddenly leaned back to do a double take. He couldn't believe what he saw lying on the counter. It was what used to be an empty milk jug, but now it had a huge watermelon inside of it. Virgil was speechless…he carefully looked around the milk jug and could not find any evidence that it had been cut or altered. Finally, he yelled down the hallway, while still keeping his eyes on the watermelon, "Hey, does anybody know how this watermelon got inside this jug?" **If you were to answer Virgil, you would say...**

____

4. You just finished touring a car manufacturing plant. The tour guide is explaining to the group that it takes 15 molding machines 15 minutes to make 15 car bumpers. After a long pause, the guide asked if anyone knew how long it would take 50 molding machines to make 50 car bumpers. **You raise your hand to answer the question and say...**_________________________________

5. Frida's daughter, Sara is running a 5k race and the winner gets a week in Paris She promised to take her mom if she won, so Frida is on the sidelines cheering her on. Suddenly she sees Sara pass the person in second place! Thrilled with excitement, she grabs her cell phone and call's her husband. As soon as he answers, she screams into the phone, **"Honey, Sara is in** ___________ **place!"**

<u>**Long Term Memory Exercise**</u>

Read the hints given for each question below to determine the names of these popular television shows.

1)   The star of this show played 'Steve Douglas', the father of three boys, Mike, Robbi and Chip. After losing his wife, who was never on the show, Steve hired a butler to do the cooking and cleaning, and did his best to raise his three sons on his own.
Name that show: ______ __________ _______

2)   The lyrics to this sitcom, which became popular in the 70's, went as follows..."Just sit right back and you'll hear a tale, a tale of a fateful trip, that started from this tropic port aboard this tiny ship.
Name that show: ______________ __________

3)   The Cartwright's owned the Ponderosa Ranch during and after the Civil War. Ben Cartwright's sons were named, Adam, Little Joe, and Hoss. (Hint: One of the sons was played by Michael Landon.)
Name that show: _________________

4)   This show was titled after the main character,'s **real** name. However, he went by Rob Petrie on the show. The name of his TV wife was Laura, played by Mary Tyler Moore. Their good friends were Buddy Sorrell and Sally Rogers. (Rob was known for tripping over the ottoman, which he did during the show's intro song.)
Name that show: ______ ________ ______ ________ _______

5)   This show aired in various versions from 1952 to 1989 and was hosted by Dick Clark. Usually airing on Saturdays, this popular show featured teenagers dancing to top 40 hits.
Name that show: _____________ _________________

6)   This game show, first hosted by Bob Barker, aired in 1972 and is still popular today. The audience is usually wildly excited, hoping their name is called and they're the next contestant on the...
Name that show: ______ _________ ____ __________

7)   Air Force captain Anthony "Tony" Nelson, played by Larry Hagman, was stranded on a desert island after his space capsule malfunctioned on re-entry. While on the island, he found an unusual bottle. As soon as he opened the bottle, a woman, played by Barbara Eden, suddenly appeared!
Name that show: ____ __________ _____ _____________

$$\begin{array}{r} \$4.92 \\ \$9.92 \\ + \ \$2.89 \\ \hline \end{array}$$

We review math skills often because math is something many of us use daily, and will continue to use throughout our lifetime. Just like any skill, if we don't use it, we risk losing it. Our goal is to provide the tools you need to retain as many skills as possible so you can age well!

Missing Variables

$$\begin{array}{r} \$1.42 \\ \$0.96 \\ + \ \$4.38 \\ \hline \end{array}$$

$13 = 26 - s$

_____

Missing Equations

$10 - \underline{\ \ } = 4$

$13 - 8 = d$

_____

$14 - \underline{\ \ } = 7$

$$\begin{array}{r} \$9.54 \\ \$7.97 \\ + \ \$1.98 \\ \hline \end{array}$$

$27 - 8 = n$

_____

$\underline{\ \ } - 2 = 9$

$6 = m - 6$

_____

$13 - \underline{\ \ } = 9$

$$\begin{array}{r} \$5.83 \\ \$6.73 \\ + \ \$3.60 \\ \hline \end{array}$$

$1 = y - 14$

_____

$\underline{\ \ } - 7 = 9$

Long Division

$$\begin{array}{r} \$7.71 \\ \$3.61 \\ + \ \$9.92 \\ \hline \end{array}$$

$22\overline{)3441}$

$71\overline{)3084}$

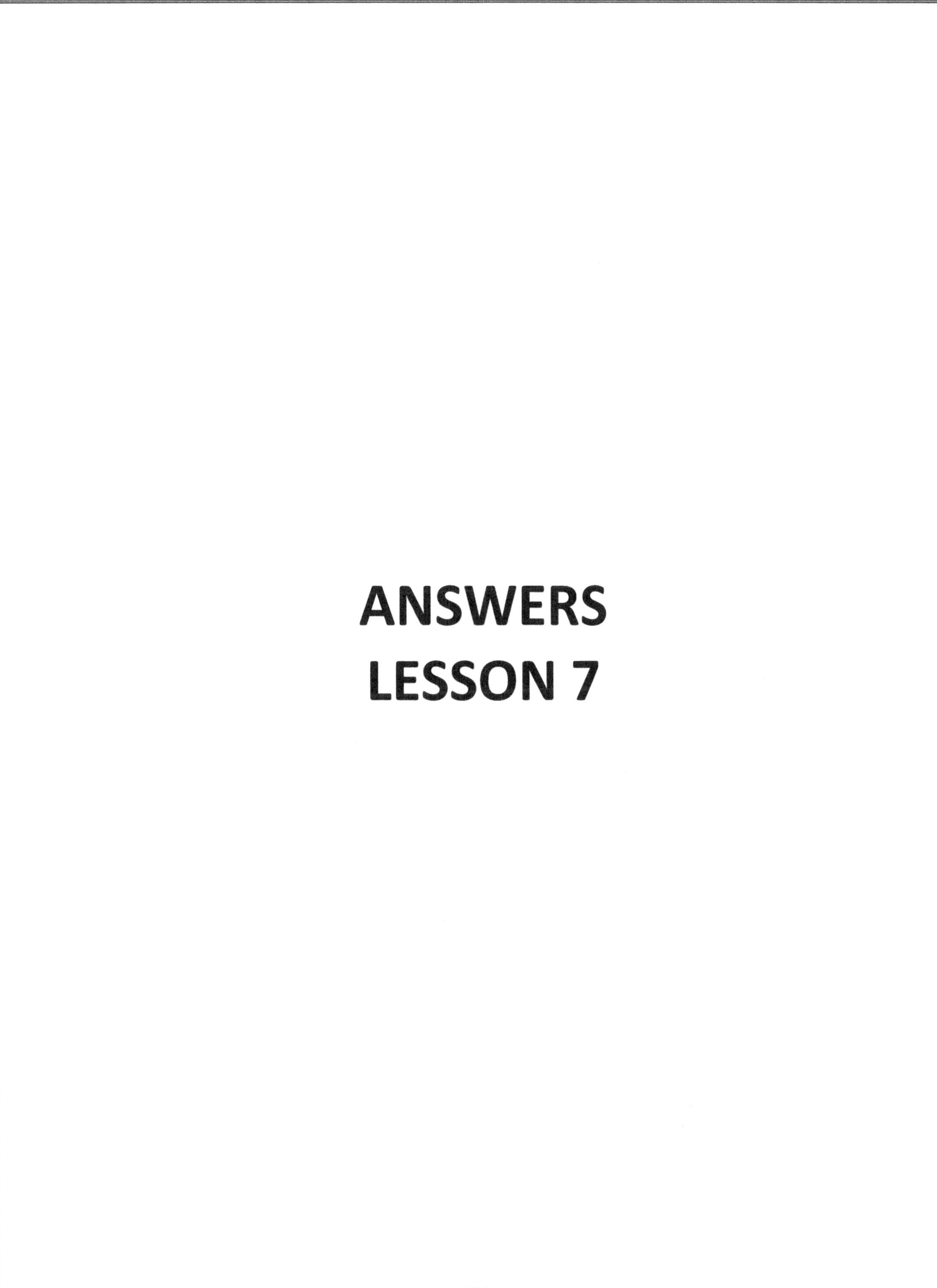

ANSWERS
LESSON 7

Answers to Lesson 7

<u>Answers to Language Vocab Centers-Attention to Detailed Instruction:</u>
Notes: Answers will vary.
<u>There are more words contained in this activity then listed below.</u>

bear	hire	meat	hare	doe	doer	mob
him	boom	hair	gut	rim	boo	bar
bare	air	moon	tag	turn	rut	game
vibe	too	toon	ear	age	tame	room

<u>Answers to Creative Thinking-Problem Solving</u>

1. Ron should find a way to put a few small <u>holes **IN** the bottom of the</u> <u>treasure chest</u> to let the sand out. (He's putting something 'IN' the chest.)
   These are the types of riddles that give your brain a great workout and strengthen your problem-solving skills.

2. The first thing Andrea should light is the **<u>MATCH.</u>**
   We have worded this challenge in such a way that the other items can easily distract you from the real answer.

3. **The watermelon was put into the empty milk jug as <u>seed</u>, and <u>then grew</u> to be a watermelon.**
   This type of brain challenge really forces your brain to think outside of the box and exercises the part of your brain that controls 'logic'.

4. **<u>It would take 50 molding machines 15 minutes to make 50 car bumpers.</u>**
   The machines require 15 minutes to make a car bumper, regardless of *how many machines are producing them, or how many car bumpers are being produced. The brain loves to take short-cuts and one way it does this is through the 'automated response system'. (What makes the most sense?) Then comes a quick answer. Sometimes this efficiency is helpful, and other times, it's not.*

5. **<u>Sarah is in 2nd place.</u>**
   This is one more example of the brain's efficiency at work. A quick 'non-reflective' response is, 'she passed the person in second, and first place is before second, so she's in first place. This is the answer most people give, with the exception of those that love to analyze questions such as these. (If Sarah passes the person in 2nd place, she's is taking her place.)

Answers to Lesson 7

Answers to Long-Term Memory Exercise

1) MY THREE SONS
2) GILLIGAN'S ISLAND
3) BONANZA
4) THE DICK VAN DYKE SHOW
5) AMERICAN BANDSTAND
6) THE PRICE IS RIGHT
7) I DREAM OF JEANNIE

Answers to Math Skills Review

Adding Money	Missing Variables	Missing Equations
$17.73	s=13	6
$6.76	d=5	7
$19.49	n=19	11
$16.16	m=12	4
$21.24	y=15	16

Long Division

```
        156 r-9
22 ⟌13441
    22
    124
    110
    141
    132
      9
```

Long Division

```
        43 r-31
71 ⟌3084
   284
   244
   213
    31
```

Use this space for drawing, doodling,
note taking.... and more

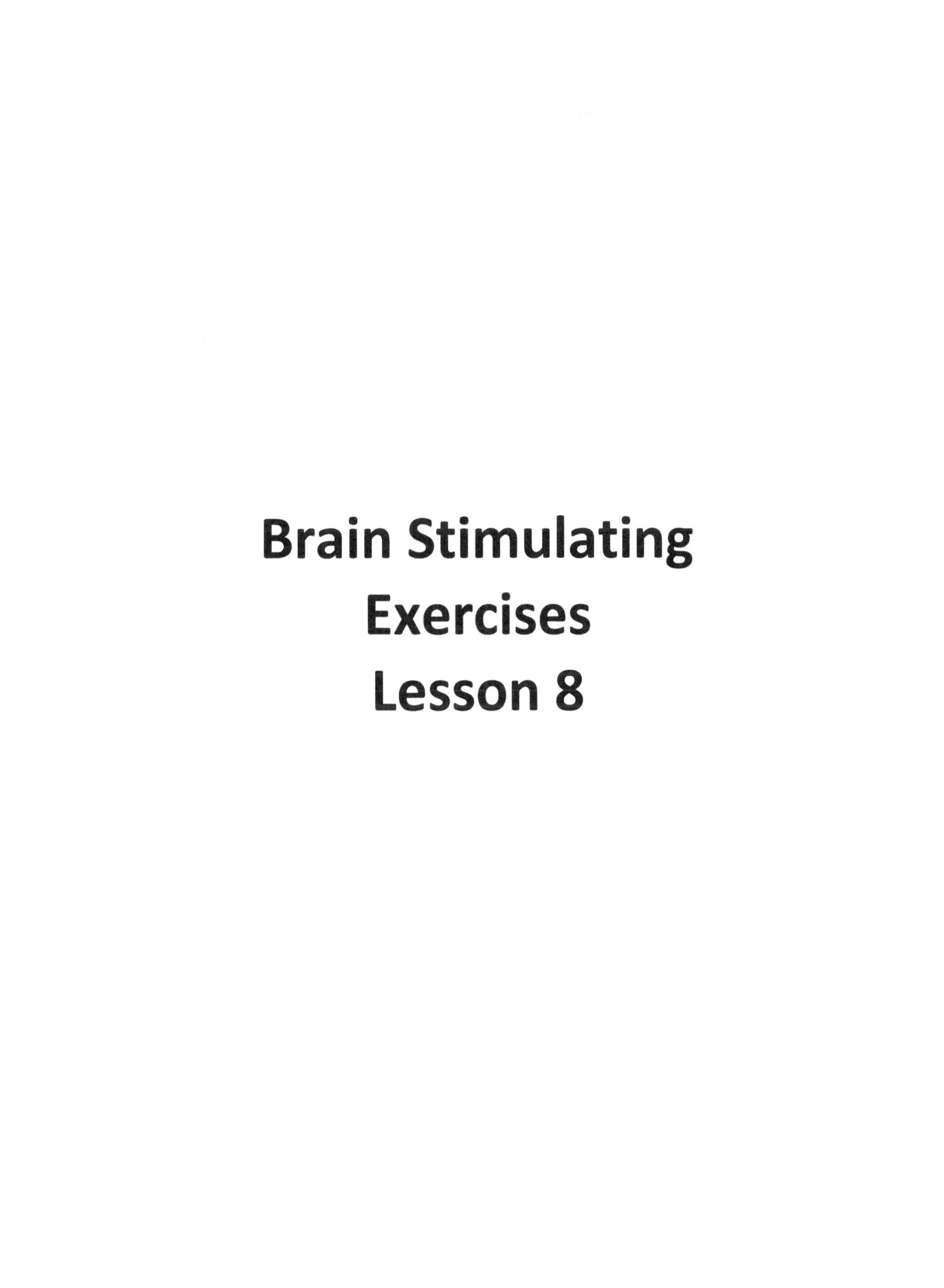

Brain Stimulating Exercises
Lesson 8

<u>Reminder Page</u>

Don't forget to check off the following after you complete them today:

____ Exercise

____ Prayer/Meditation

____ Self-Affirmations

SELF-AFFIRMATIONS

I WILL BE FULL OF JOY TODAY.

HAPPINESS WILL BE ONE OF MY HIGHEST PRIORITIES.

I AM BRAVE AND FEAR WILL NOT HOLD ME BACK.

I WILL ACCEPT WHAT I CANNOT CHANGE.

I WILL DO MY BEST TO CHANGE THE THINGS I DON'T LIKE.

<u>LESSON 8:</u> Things You Can Do for Your Brain

1)   <u>Sleeping</u>: Many different things can interrupt deep sleep and/or interfere with REM sleep, and both deep sleep and REM sleep are necessary for good mental health. Healthy sleep patterns contribute to better learning and retention and also benefit the brain's memory center. Research studies have shown that not getting enough sleep reduces the amount of gray matter in the frontal lobe.
(This isn't a good thing.)

The frontal lobe is the area of the brain that supports working memory and executive functioning. These areas are extremely important because they're needed to perform the tasks we do every day.

2) <u>Eating the Right Foods</u>: Research continues to confirm the impact healthy food can have on both the brain and the body. For example, foods high in antioxidants are vital to a healthy immune system, which is why we should regularly include them in our diet.

Here are just a few suggestions:

Nuts , such as almonds or pecans, (if no allergies),
   blueberries, raspberries, avocados, tomatoes,
Keep in mind, if a certain food is good for your body, it's also beneficial to your brain, (and your mind).

3) <u>Brain Stimulating Activities</u>: Keeping the brain challenged has been shown in countless research studies to help prevent the loss of gray matter in the brain. (This IS a good thing.) Creative problem solving, drawing, and writing poetry are just a few of the many ways we can stretch the mind and exercise the brain.

4) <u>Stay Positive</u>: Remember…you don't have to sit and ponder on every thought that comes into your mind. You can use self-control to counter negative thoughts by replacing them with positive ones. Research now shows that consistent negative thinking has a negative impact on the brain and body.

RESOURCE:
Zimmer, C. (2014, June 20). This is Your Brain on Writing . Retrieved from New York Times:
https://www.nytimes.com/2014/06/19/science/researching-the-brain-o

Poetry is a form of expression. Research reveals that exercising our creative side can open our mind to possibilities that lead to the most innovative ideas.

Below are two short poems, both very different. Keep in mind, there are all types of poetry… some funny, some serious, some rhyme, and some seem free of any form. It's simply a way to express ourselves.

Carefully read poem #1.

Poem #1   There was a gal named Mary, she married Jerry DeBary.
Each time that he drank dairy, he was rude and quite contrary,
He'd say things like, "you're hairy", which made Mary quite weary.
So she went out to the prairie, and found some 'special' berries,
And instead of serving dairy, she served Jerry the berries.
He ate them all, though leery, And now there's no more Jerry.

1. What do you think of the Poem #1?_______________________________

____

____

Next, read poem #2 then answer the questions below.

Poem #2   What is this thing I often feel, I struggle to describe,
It lies below within a pit, so far down deep inside.
Is it pain, discontentment, maybe fear or pride?
I wish that it would flee this place, just shrivel up and die,
And in the empty space it leaves, that joy there would abide.

1. What do you think about this poem? _____________________

____

____

2. What feelings do you think the author was trying to express? _____________

____

3. Does the poem stir up any feelings or emotions as you read it?

____

____

When you are finished, use the following page to write two poems of your own. Remember, poetry doesn't have to rhyme. It can be funny, serious, or even somewhat nonsensical. You can allow your poetry to express your current mood or change it up. Just let your inhibitions go and challenge your creativity.

Writing plays an important role in brain function, so write as often as you can.

POETRY-A FORM OF EXPRESSION

As you write your poetry, keep in mind that the purpose for writing can be altruistic, educational, inspirational, therapeutic or just for fun. Before you begin, here are a few more outcomes we can experience when we engage in various types of poetry.

1. People who write poetry exercise their insight and sensitivity in profound ways.
2. Poetry provides a safe and private experience, with individual control over the outcome.
3. Poetry provides a basis to improve our personal communication, especially regarding personal issues, and can help you build stronger relationships.
4. People who write poetry use a variety of cognitive skills and can increase their language and vocabulary skills as well.
5. People who write poetry can become more in touch with various issues of life, and has a way of increasing the meaning of life to them, while developing a more spiritual appreciation of life.

1. ON THE LINES BELOW, WRITE EITHER A SERIOUS POEM OR A FUN POEM ON THE SUBJECT OF **'THE FOREST'**

____

____

____

____

____

____

____

WorksCited

Benefits of Writing Poetry. (2009). Retrieved from Pongo Teen Writing : https://www.pongoteenwriting.org/Benefits-of-Writing-Poetry.html

REVIEW: Language Center-Synonyms

Exercise your language skills by circling the word that has the closest meaning to the word in **bold**.

1. Zack asked his personal trainer if he could help him get his 'beach body' back within three months. To which the personal trainer replied, "***affirmative*** sir".

    a. negative   b. planning   c. agreement

2. As Brooke left the store, she got on the escalator and began her ***descent.***

    a. downward   b. lateral   c. good

3. Cristan felt very ***melancholy*** as she sat by the window watching the birds.

    a. sad   b. anxious   c. frightened

4. Jake believes everyone should ***volunteer*** to help in the community.

    a. reject   b. offer   c. agree

5. Nick was ***inundated*** with checks from his renters.

    a. punctuated   b. underwhelmed   c. flooded

6. Tanner and Tukker were glad they didn't live under a ***dictatorship.***

    a. republic   b. tyranny   c. changeable

7. Ken and Mel engage in ***moderate*** exercise each week.

    a. timely   b. excessive   c. average

8. Judy had been traveling for hours, so she decided to pull over and rest in a ***vacant*** parking lot.

    a. occupied   b. adjacent   c. empty

9. Ruth's ***discernment*** was helpful in her career as a marriage counselor.

    a. uncertainty   b. probable   c. insight

10. Donna and Glenna were determined to ***engage*** the enemy.

    a. confront   b. offer   c. surrender

Exercise: Maintaining Math/Geometry Skills

456,483,276
+767,618,754

549,199,857
+687,962,184

763,377,967
+848,932,294

564,873,786
+879,246,619

867,868,492
+546,747,898

1.   What percentage of the circle above is missing?____________

2.   What percentage of the circle above is remaining? __________

3.   In fractions, approximately what portion of the circle above is gray? __________

4.   In fractions, approximately what portion of the circle above is white? __________

QUICK REVIEW

5.   An 'OCTAGON' has ______sides?

6.   A 'PENTAGON' has ______sides?

Draw these 2 shapes in the space below.

ANSWERS
LESSON 8

Answers to Lesson 8

Answers to Poetry Activities

Answers will vary according to individual opinions and thoughts

Answers to Language Center-Synonyms

1. c-agreement
2. a-downward
3. a-sad
4. b-offer
5. c-flooded
6. b-tyranny
7. c-average
8. c-empty
9. c-insight
10. a-confront

Answers to Math-Geometry-Percentage Review

Answers to Addition Problems

1,224,102,030

1,237,162,041

1,612,310,261

1,444,120,405

1,414,616,390

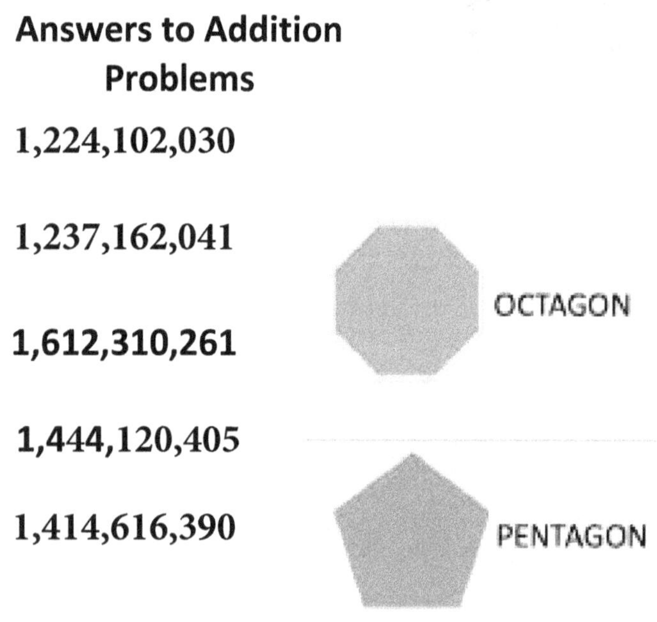

1. 25% of the circle is missing

2. 75% of the circle remains

3. Approximately 1/4 of the circle is gray

4. Approximately 3/4 of the circle is white

5. An 'Octagon has 8 sides

6. A 'Pentagon has 5 sides

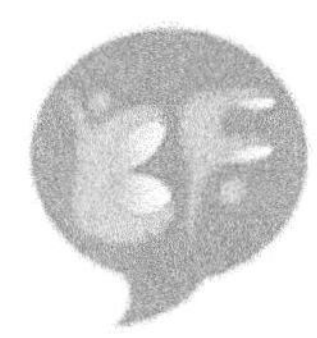

Congratulations!

You have completed the next level of 'The Aging Well' Program

The BrainFlex System
The Whole Person Approach to Brain Health

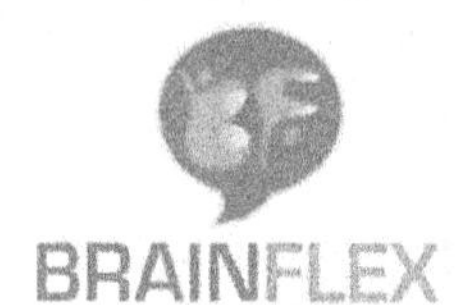

Personal Action Plan
&
Wellness Notes
Guide

The 'Personal Action Plan' is designed for monthly use and can be used along side your BrainFlex workbook.

The 'Personal Action Plan' allows you to set goals for each of the four major concepts included in the BrainFlex system, (key components to aging well).

 The 'Weekly Wellness Notes' provide a way for you to track your progress towards those goals.

This is not only a great way to hold yourself accountable, it's also a wonderful resource for families and doctors, as it allows them to read about your day to day activities and see, first hand, your strong commitment to aging well.

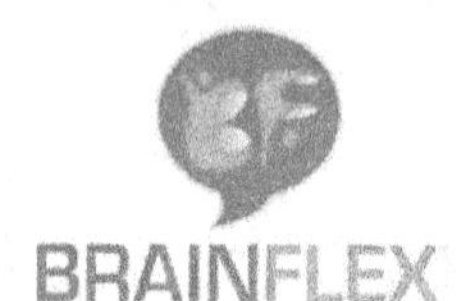

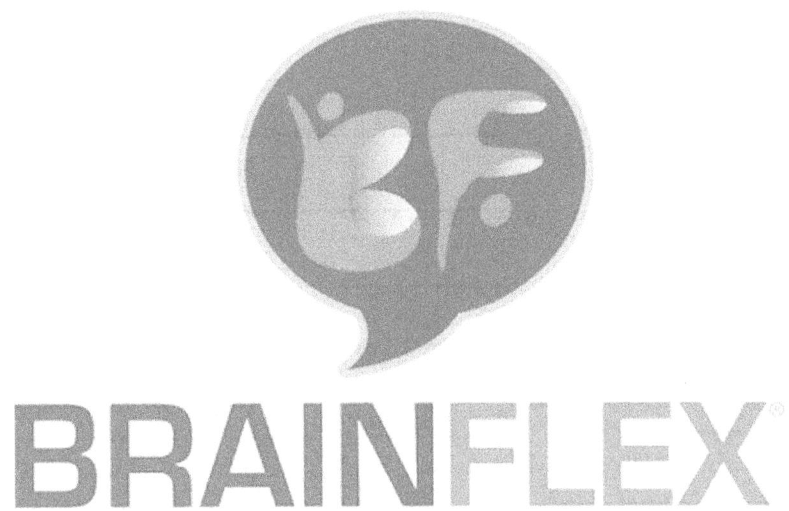

Personal
Action Plan

(one month)

<u>SOCIALIZATION</u>

| Goal #1 | Steps I will take to achieve goal #1 |
| Goal #2 | Steps I will take to achieve goal #2 |

<u>NUTRITION</u>

| Goal #1 | Steps I will take to achieve goal #1 |
| Goal #2 | Steps I will take to achieve goal #2 |

Rate your current stress level management on a scale from
1-10 (10 being the best) _________
What steps can you take to improve this number? _________________
____
____

Goal #1	Steps I will take to achieve goal #1
________________________	__________________________________
________________________	__________________________________
________________________	__________________________________
Goal #2	Steps I will take to achieve goal #2
________________________	__________________________________
________________________	__________________________________
________________________	__________________________________

EXERCISE

Goal #1	Steps I will take to achieve goal #1
________________________	__________________________________
________________________	__________________________________
________________________	__________________________________
Goal #2	Steps I will take to achieve goal #2
________________________	__________________________________
________________________	__________________________________
________________________	__________________________________

Rate your current sleep patterns this month on a scale from
1-10 (10 being the best) _________
What can you do to improve in this area? _______________
____

Watch for correlations between your sleep patterns and how often you engage in the BrainFlex concepts.

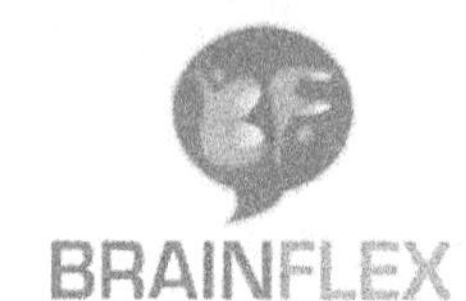

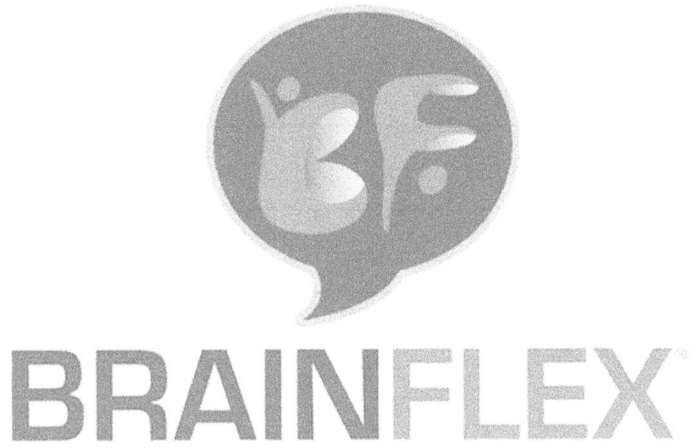

Wellness Journaling
Week 1

These journaling pages have been included in this workbook
in order for you to track the successful steps you're taking
each week towards the goals you've written in your
'Action Plan'.
At the end of each week, take a few minutes
to jot down some notes about your aging
well journey on the following pages.

Wellness Journaling: Tracking progress toward 'Action Plan' Goals

<u>Socialization:</u> How have I strengthened my social connections this week?

1.____

2.____

3.____

4.____

5.____

6.____

7.____

<u>Nutrition:</u> Healthy foods I incorporated into my diet this week:

1.____

2.____

3.____

4.____

5.____

6.____

7.____

In order to manage my stress this week, I engaged in the following...

______________ ______________ ______________

______________ ______________ ______________

BrainFlex® Wellness©

Wellness Journaling: Tracking progress toward 'Action Plan' Goals

<u>**Brain Training:**</u> Brain stimulating activities I engaged in this week:

1.____

2.____

3.____

4.____

5.____

6.____

7.____

<u>**Exercise:**</u> I participated in the following exercises this week:

1.____

2.____

3.____

4.____

5.____

6.____

7.____

On a scale from 1 to 10, (10 being the best), how well did I sleep this week?

Monday: ___________ Tuesday:_________ Wednesday: __________

Thursday: ___________ Friday: ___________

Was there a correlation between how I slept and the ways in which I engaged in the above areas? _______________________________

____

BrainFlex® Wellness©

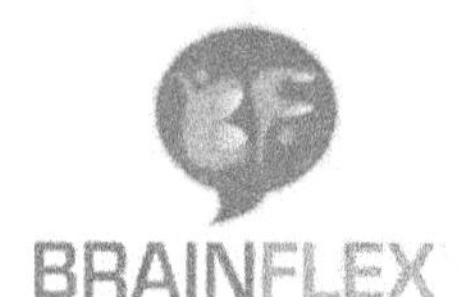

BRAINFLEX

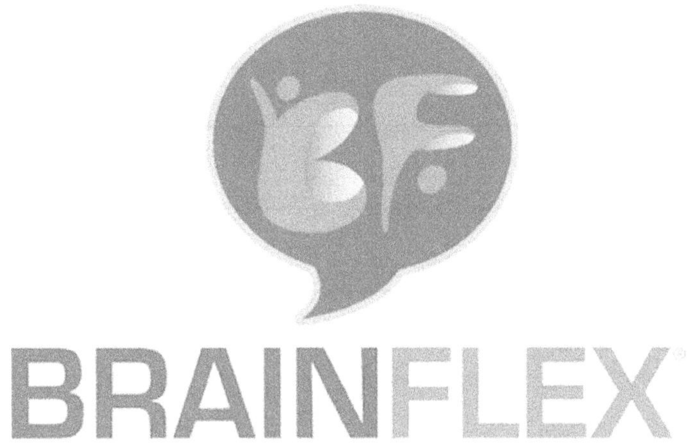

Wellness Journaling
Week 2

These journaling pages have been included in this workbook
in order for you to track the successful steps you're taking
each week towards the goals you've written in your
'Action Plan'.
At the end of each week, take a few minutes
to jot down some notes about your aging
well journey on the following pages.

Wellness Journaling: Tracking progress toward 'Action Plan' Goals

<u>Socialization:</u> How have I strengthened my social connections this week?

1.____

2.____

3.____

4.____

5.____

6.____

7.____

<u>Nutrition:</u> Healthy foods I incorporated into my diet this week:

1.____

2.____

3.____

4.____

5.____

6.____

7.____

In order to manage my stress this week, I engaged in the following...

____________________ ____________________ ____________________

____________________ ____________________ ____________________

BrainFlex® Wellness©

Wellness Journaling: Tracking progress toward 'Action Plan' Goals

<u>**Brain Training:**</u> Brain stimulating activities I engaged in this week:

1.____

2.____

3.____

4.____

5.____

6.____

7.____

<u>Exercise:</u> I participated in the following exercises this week:

1.____

2.____

3.____

4.____

5.____

6.____

7.____

On a scale from 1 to 10, (10 being the best), how well did I sleep this week?

Monday: ______________ Tuesday:______________ Wednesday: ______________

Thursday: ______________ Friday: ______________

Was there a correlation between how I slept and the ways in which I engaged in the above areas? ____

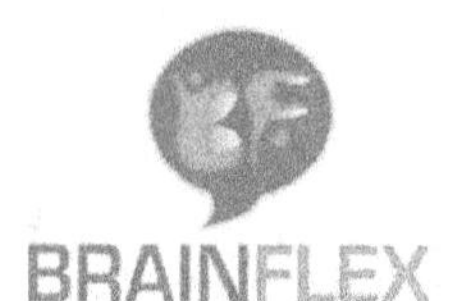

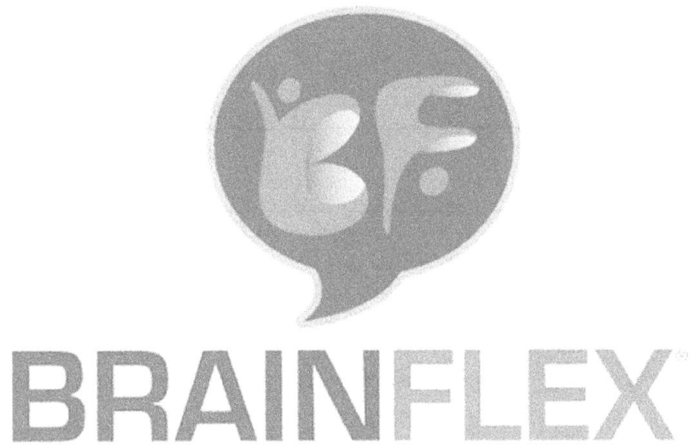

Wellness Journaling
Week 3

These journaling pages have been included in this workbook
in order for you to track the successful steps you're taking
each week towards the goals you've written in your
'Action Plan'.
At the end of each week, take a few minutes
to jot down some notes about your aging
well journey on the following pages.

Wellness Journaling: Tracking progress toward 'Action Plan' Goals

<u>Socialization</u>: How have I strengthened my social connections this week?

1.____

2.____

3.____

4.____

5.____

6.____

7.____

<u>Nutrition</u>: Healthy foods I incorporated into my diet this week:

1.____

2.____

3.____

4.____

5.____

6.____

7.____

In order to manage my stress this week, I engaged in the following...

______________ ______________ ______________

______________ ______________ ______________

Wellness Journaling: Tracking progress toward 'Action Plan' Goals

<u>**Brain Training:**</u> Brain stimulating activities I engaged in this week:

1.____

2.____

3.____

4.____

5.____

6.____

7.____

<u>**Exercise:**</u> I participated in the following exercises this week:

1.____

2.____

3.____

4.____

5.____

6.____

7.____

On a scale from 1 to 10, (10 being the best), how well did I sleep this week?

Monday: _____________ Tuesday:___________ Wednesday: ____________

Thursday: ___________ Friday: ___________

Was there a correlation between how I slept and the ways in which I engaged in the above areas? __________________________________

____

BrainFlex® Wellness©

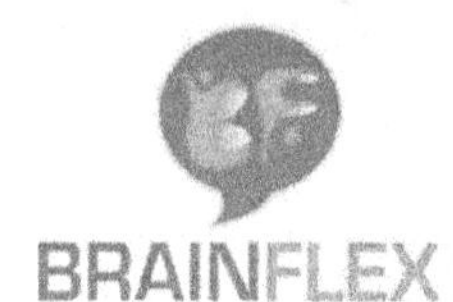

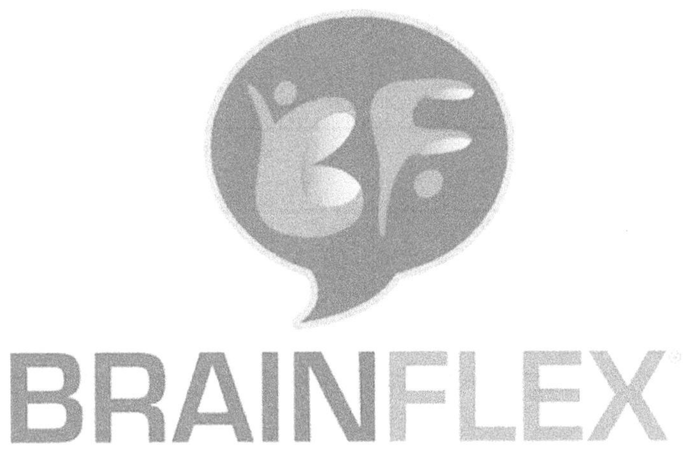

Wellness Journaling
Week 4

These journaling pages have been included in this workbook
in order for you to track the successful steps you're taking
each week towards the goals you've written in your
'Action Plan'.
At the end of each week, take a few minutes
to jot down some notes about your aging
well journey on the following pages.

Wellness Journaling: Tracking progress toward 'Action Plan' Goals

<u>Socialization:</u> How have I strengthened my social connections this week?

1.____

2.____

3.____

4.____

5.____

6.____

7.____

<u>Nutrition:</u> Healthy foods I incorporated into my diet this week:

1.____

2.____

3.____

4.____

5.____

6.____

7.____

In order to manage my stress this week, I engaged in the following...

__________________ __________________ __________________

__________________ __________________ __________________

Wellness Journaling: Tracking progress toward 'Action Plan' Goals

Brain Training: Brain stimulating activities I engaged in this week:

1.____

2.____

3.____

4.____

5.____

6.____

7.____

Exercise: I participated in the following exercises this week:

1.____

2.____

3.____

4.____

5.____

6.____

7.____

On a scale from 1 to 10, (10 being the best), how well did I sleep this week?
Monday: ______________ Tuesday:____________ Wednesday: ____________
Thursday: ____________ Friday: ____________
Was there a correlation between how I slept and the ways in which I engaged in the above areas? __________________________________ ____

BrainFlex® Wellness©

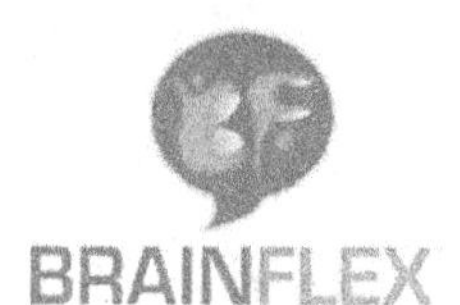

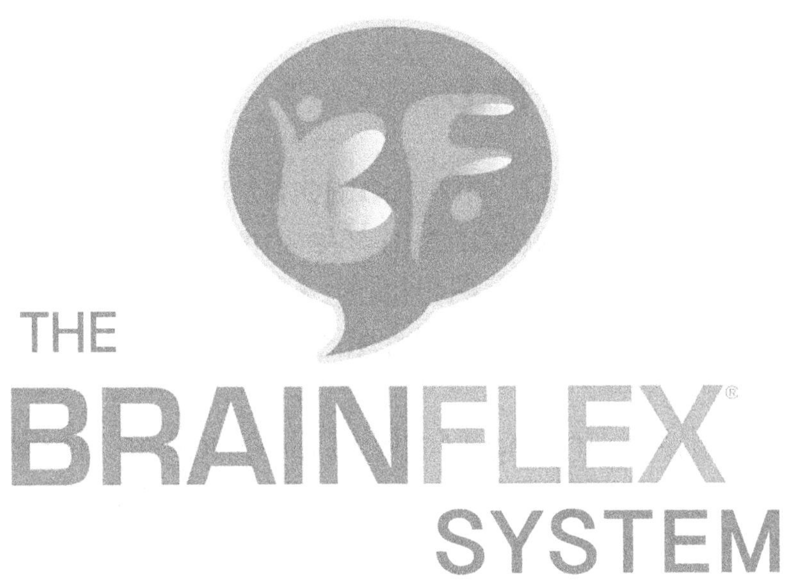

ABOUT
US

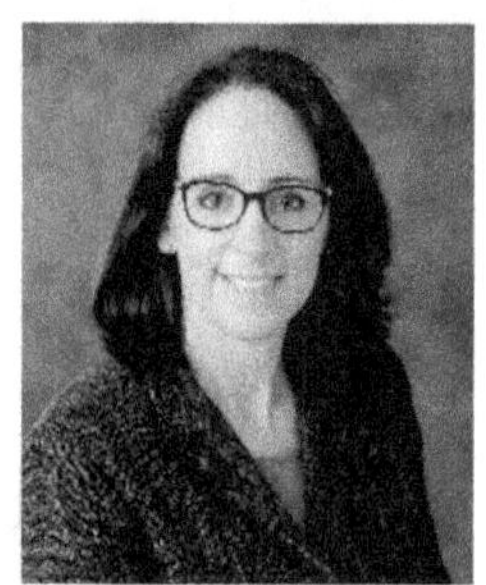

Rosemary D. Laird, M.D.

Rosemary D. Laird, M.D., graduated from Georgetown University School of Medicine in Washington, D.C. She completed a Fellowship in Geriatric Medicine and earned a Masters in Healthcare Administration.

Dr. Laird was the founding Medical Director of 'Health First Aging Services' and 'The Center for Family Caregivers' in Melbourne, Florida. She then led the development of the Memory Disorder Clinic for Advent Health Maturing Minds program in Orlando, Florida.

For over 20 years, Dr. Laird has provided specialty care for people with Alzheimer's disease and related disorders. She has been recognized as a Space Coast Humanitarian in 2011 and received the American Geriatrics Society's Clinician of the Year award in 2013.

Currently Dr. Laird is pursuing her dream of providing a new and innovative 'support system' for families facing challenges related to cognitive concerns. Check out NAN,
(Navigating Aging Needs), at **https://nanforcaregivers.com**

Rosemary Laird, M.D., is a Geriatrician and recognized expert in diagnosing and caring for patients with Alzheimer's disease.
She is an advocate for the support of family caregivers and co-authored the book Take Your Oxygen First: Preserving Your Health and Happiness While Caring for a loved one with Alzheimer's Disease.

Melissa Arnold, Founder of The BrainFlex® System
www.brainflexwellness.com

Melissa began working with seniors in 2009, as the director of an adult day program in Michigan. After moving to Orlando in 2010, she continued working in the senior care industry as a consultant, advising seniors in need of assistance in the home. Eventually, with a desire to improve the quality of care her clients received, she moved into Human Resources where she focused on recruiting caregivers who had a heart for seniors. As the Director of Human Resources, Melissa also focused on agency compliance related to AHCA and Joint Commission regulations as well as state and federal labor laws. In addition, Melissa provided on-going training for employees and education for the families of her clients. After restructuring this part of the business, Melissa was offered the position of Director of Operations, where she focused on aligning the systems and process within the business in order to provide the very best customer and employee experience. The next step for Melissa was the position of 'Executive Director', which included oversight of the Nursing Department, Human Resources, Operations, and training and development of the Sales and Marketing team. As Executive Director, Melissa led a team of directors with a focus on business development while remaining intentional in her mission to invest in the lives of her employees.

In August of 2018, Melissa made the difficult decision to resign as Executive Director of Senior Helpers in order to focus on BrainFlex Wellness Club, which she had founded in 2015. The idea for BrainFlex began in 2014, when Melissa noticed an increase in seniors experiencing dementia. It was at this time, she became a researcher of researchers, determined to find the various ways in which seniors could be proactive against age-related diseases. Her research consistently revealed the following key areas: exercise, nutrition, brain stimulating activities, social connections, prayer/meditation and sleep, as well as stress management and maintaining a positive mindset.

Once Covid-19 hit the world, Melissa began to pivot her business, offering BrainFlex sessions on-line while moving the curriculum into a series of workbooks, now referred to as The BrainFlex System. Each of the three workbook series' are designed for a specific cognitive level, with a focus on engaging the 'whole person'. Many doctors and healthcare professionals strongly encourage their patients and clients to utilize the BrainFlex system, and now we're excited to make our interactive workbooks available to seniors everywhere.

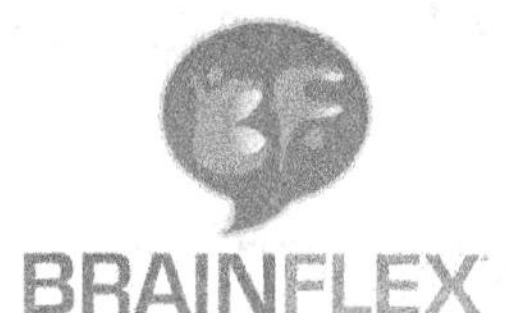

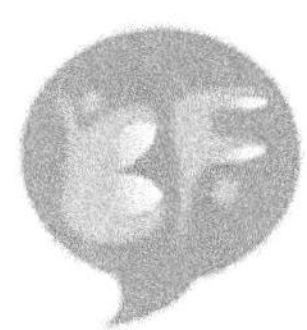

To order or reorder the next BrainFlex Workbook,

or to order one of our 'Wisdom Journals',
choose one of the following options:

1.) Order through the BrainFlex Wellness website.
www.brainflexwellness.com

Once you're there, click on the 'WORKBOOK' tab.

On this page you will be given two choices.

A.) Order directly from amazon

B.) Save 20% by ordering directly from the

BrainFlex online store.

Click on the option you prefer and follow the step by
step instructions.

2.) As an alternative to the above choices, you may also
send us an email requesting which series and volume(s)
you would like to order, along with the number of
workbooks you would like. Please send your request to:

marnold@brainflexwellness.com

NOTE: Type 'WORKBOOK ORDER' or 'WORKBOOK
REORDER' in the subject line.

Once we receive your request, we will send an invoice to
your email and you can pay the amount due on line,
directly from the invoice. Your workbooks will be
ordered and on the way once we receive 'notice of
payment'.

www.ingramcontent.com/pod-product-compliance
Lightning Source LLC
Chambersburg PA
CBHW081414250726
48654CB00013B/1699